AI
in
Healthcare

By
Tantrajnana Vedike

©Copyrights: Tantrajnana

Preface

Welcome to the forefront of healthcare innovation, where the convergence of artificial intelligence (AI) and medicine is revolutionizing the way we understand, diagnose, and treat illnesses. This book explores the profound impact of AI technologies on modern healthcare, offering a comprehensive journey through its applications, challenges, and transformative potential.

In recent years, AI has emerged as a powerful tool in healthcare, capable of analyzing vast amounts of data with unprecedented speed and accuracy. From interpreting medical imaging scans to personalizing treatment plans based on genetic profiles, AI is reshaping every facet of the medical field. This transformation promises not only to enhance clinical decision-making but also to improve patient outcomes and operational efficiency across healthcare systems globally.

The chapters within this book delve into diverse aspects of AI in healthcare, highlighting real-world examples and case studies from leading institutions and companies at the forefront of this technological revolution. We explore how AI-driven innovations are accelerating drug discovery, predicting patient outcomes, optimizing hospital workflows, and enabling more precise surgical interventions.

However, amidst these advancements lie critical considerations of ethics, privacy, and the equitable distribution of AI benefits. As AI continues to integrate deeper into healthcare, navigating these ethical landscapes becomes paramount to ensuring responsible and inclusive implementation.

Through this exploration, we aim to provide healthcare professionals, researchers, policymakers, and enthusiasts with a comprehensive understanding of AI's current capabilities and future potential in transforming medicine. Whether you are a seasoned practitioner or a curious observer, this book invites you to embark on a journey into the promising yet complex intersection of AI and healthcare.

Join us as we unravel the possibilities of AI in healthcare and envision a future where technology not only complements but also elevates the practice of medicine, ultimately advancing the well-being of patients worldwide.

Table of Contents

Sl. No	Topics	Page No.
1.	**Introduction to AI in Healthcare**	1
1.1	Historical Evolution and Milestones of AI in Medicine	6
1.2	Overview of AI Technologies in Healthcare	11
2.	**AI in Medical Imaging and Diagnostics**	16
2.1	AI Algorithms for Image Analysis and Interpretation	22
2.2	Applications of AI in Radiology and Pathology	31
2.3	Enhancing Diagnostic Accuracy with Machine Learning	37
3.	**AI in Predictive Analytics and Disease Prevention**	42
3.1	Predictive Modeling for Disease Outbreaks	48
3.2	AI in Personalized Medicine and Risk Assessment	54

	3.3	Early Detection and Prevention Strategies using AI	60
4.		**AI in Treatment and Patient Care**	**65**
	4.1	AI-driven Treatment Planning and Recommendations	71
	4.2	Virtual Health Assistants and Chatbots	76
	4.3	AI in Remote Monitoring and Telehealth	82
5.		**AI in Drug Discovery and Development**	**88**
	5.1	Accelerating Drug Discovery with AI	93
	5.2	AI in Clinical Trials and Research	98
	5.3	Personalized Drug Development and Precision Medicine	103
6.		**AI in Healthcare Operations and Management**	**109**
	6.1	AI in Healthcare Supply Chain Management	115
	6.2	AI for Workforce Management and Scheduling	121

	6.3	AI in Healthcare warehouse and storage management	127
7.	**AI in Genomics and Bioinformatics**		**132**
	7.1	AI in Genetic Sequencing and Analysis	138
	7.2	Applications of AI in Personalized Genomics	144
	7.3	AI-driven Insights in Bioinformatics	150
8.	**Ethical and Legal Considerations of AI in Healthcare**		**156**
	8.1	Ethical Implications of AI in Medicine	159
	8.2	Privacy and Security Concerns	163
	8.3	Regulatory and Legal Frameworks for AI in Healthcare	167
9.	**Implementation and Integration of AI in Healthcare Systems**		**171**
	9.1	Strategies for Successful AI Implementation	175
	9.2	Integration of AI with Existing Healthcare Systems	179
	9.3	AI in Electronic Health Records (EHRs)	182

	9.4	Overcoming Challenges in AI Adoption	188
10.		**Future Trends and Innovations in AI Healthcare**	**192**
	10.1	Emerging AI Technologies and Innovations	197
	10.2	The Future of AI in Global Health	203
	10.3	Addressing Future Challenges and Opportunities	211
11.		**Real-world Case Study Examples**	**214**
	11.1	Case Study 1: Historical Evolution and Milestones of AI in Medicine by IBM Watson Health	214
	11.2	Case Study 2: AI in Medical Imaging and Diagnostics in Healthcare at San Francisco (UCSF) Medical Center, USA	217
	11.3	Case Study 3: AI in Predictive Analytics and Disease Prevention at Cleveland Clinic, USA	220
	11.4	Case Study 4: Virtual Health Assistants and Chatbots by Babylon Health	223

11.5	Case Study 5: AI in Drug Discovery and Development at Insilico Medicine	226
11.6	Case Study 6: AI in Healthcare Operations and Management at Mount Sinai Health System, USA	229
11.7	Case Study 7: AI in Genomics and Bioinformatics in Healthcare at Illumina, Inc.	232
11.8	Case Study 8: Privacy and Security Concerns for AI in Healthcare at Memorial Sloan Kettering Cancer Center, USA	235
11.9	Case Study 9: Overcoming Challenges in AI Adoption in Healthcare at Mount Sinai Health System, USA	238
11.10	11.10 Case Study 10: Future Trends and Innovations in AI Healthcare at Cleveland Clinic, USA	241
12.	**Popular Software, Applications, Platforms and Tools in AI Powered Healthcare**	**244**

1. Introduction to AI in Healthcare

Artificial Intelligence (AI) is revolutionizing the healthcare industry, offering transformative capabilities that enhance patient care, streamline operations, and drive medical innovation.

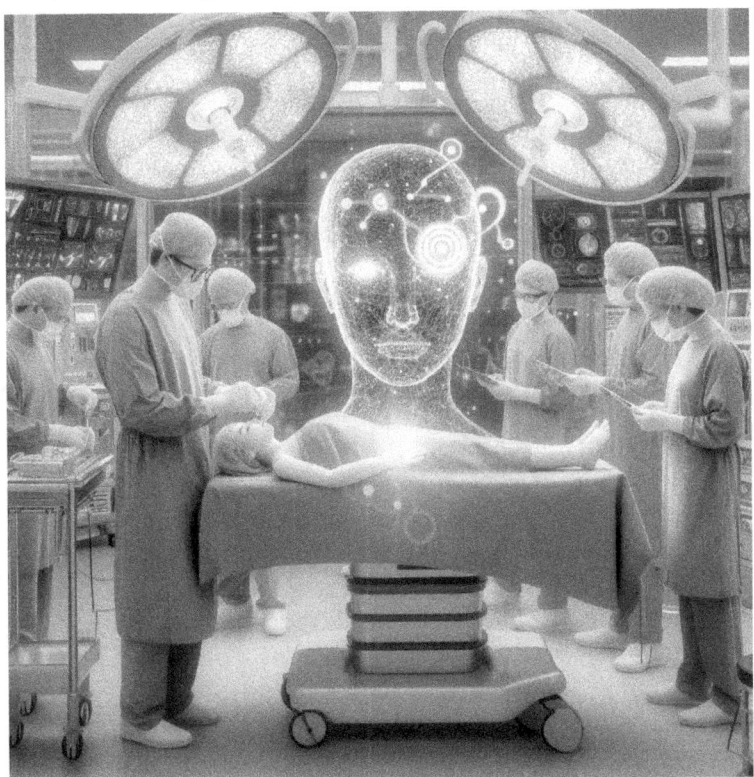

Here are key reasons why AI adoption is crucial for healthcare:

1. **Enhanced Diagnostic Accuracy:** AI-powered diagnostic tools are capable of analyzing vast amounts of patient data, including medical images, genomic data, and electronic health records (EHRs). Machine learning algorithms can detect patterns and anomalies that may not be apparent to human clinicians, leading to more accurate and timely diagnoses. For example, AI in radiology can assist in detecting tumors or abnormalities in medical scans with high precision.

2. **Personalized Treatment Planning:** AI enables personalized medicine by analyzing patient data to tailor treatment plans based on individual characteristics, such as genetic makeup, medical history, and lifestyle factors. Natural language processing (NLP) algorithms can extract valuable insights from unstructured clinical notes, helping clinicians make informed decisions about treatment options and interventions.

3. **Operational Efficiency and Workflow Automation:** AI streamlines healthcare operations by automating routine administrative tasks, such as scheduling appointments, processing billing, and managing medical records. This automation reduces administrative burden on healthcare providers, allowing them to focus more on patient care and less on paperwork. AI-powered systems can also optimize hospital workflows by predicting patient admission rates, resource allocation, and staffing needs.

4. **Drug Discovery and Development:** AI accelerates drug discovery processes by analyzing vast datasets to identify potential drug candidates and predict their efficacy and safety profiles. Machine learning models can analyze molecular structures, pharmacological data, and clinical trial results to expedite the development of new therapies for various diseases and conditions.

5. **Telemedicine and Remote Patient Monitoring:** AI technologies support telemedicine initiatives by enabling remote consultations, diagnosis, and monitoring of patients. AI-powered chatbots and virtual assistants can provide personalized healthcare information, triage patients based on symptoms, and offer guidance on self-care practices. Remote patient monitoring devices equipped with AI algorithms can continuously analyze patient data, alerting healthcare providers to potential health issues in real-time.

6. **Predictive Analytics for Preventive Healthcare:** AI facilitates predictive analytics by analyzing population health data to identify at-risk patients and predict disease

outbreaks. Machine learning models can analyze trends in patient data to forecast healthcare needs, improve vaccination strategies, and implement preventive interventions that reduce the burden of chronic diseases.

7. **Ethical Considerations in AI-driven Healthcare:** The adoption of AI in healthcare raises ethical considerations related to patient privacy, data security, and algorithm bias. Ensuring the confidentiality and integrity of patient data, addressing biases in AI algorithms that may disproportionately affect certain patient groups, and maintaining transparency in AI-driven decision-making processes are critical to fostering trust and ethical use of AI in healthcare.

8. **Future Directions and Innovation:** Looking ahead, AI continues to drive innovation in healthcare with advancements in robotics, virtual reality (VR), and augmented reality (AR) technologies. AI-powered surgical robots enhance precision and minimize invasiveness in surgical procedures, while VR and AR applications support medical training, patient education, and rehabilitation therapies.

In summary, the adoption of AI in healthcare holds immense promise for improving patient outcomes, operational efficiency, and medical innovation. By leveraging AI technologies, healthcare organizations can enhance diagnostic accuracy, personalize treatment plans, automate workflows, and advance preventive healthcare initiatives. Embracing AI-driven solutions enables healthcare providers to deliver more effective, accessible, and patient-centered care in the evolving healthcare landscape.

Examples:

AI for Enhanced Diagnostic Accuracy

Company: Aidoc

Example: Aidoc uses AI algorithms to analyze medical imaging scans (such as CT scans and MRIs) to assist radiologists in detecting abnormalities like intracranial hemorrhages or pulmonary embolisms with greater accuracy and speed.

AI for Personalized Treatment Planning

Company: Tempus

Example: Tempus utilizes AI to analyze clinical and molecular data from patients to personalize cancer treatment plans. By integrating genomic sequencing and AI analytics, Tempus helps oncologists tailor therapies based on individual genetic profiles and treatment responses.

AI for Operational Efficiency and Workflow Automation

Company: Olive

Example: Olive AI automates repetitive administrative tasks in healthcare facilities. It integrates with existing systems to streamline operations such as patient scheduling, insurance verification, and billing, improving efficiency and reducing human error.

AI in Drug Discovery and Development

Company: Insilico Medicine

Example: Insilico Medicine uses AI for drug discovery by employing deep learning to analyze biological data and predict potential drug candidates. AI-driven simulations accelerate the process of identifying molecules that could be effective in treating diseases like cancer or Alzheimer's.

AI in Telemedicine and Remote Patient Monitoring

Company: 98point6

Example: 98point6 provides AI-powered telemedicine services where patients can consult with doctors via a smartphone app. AI algorithms assist in triaging patients, conducting initial assessments, and monitoring chronic conditions remotely, enhancing access to healthcare services.

Predictive Analytics for Preventive Healthcare

Company: EarlySense

Example: EarlySense uses AI-driven analytics to monitor patients' vital signs and detect early signs of deterioration in hospital settings. By predicting patient outcomes and alerting healthcare providers to potential issues, EarlySense aids in preventive interventions and improving patient safety.

AI for Ethical Considerations in AI-driven Healthcare

Company: Google Health

Example: Google Health faces ethical considerations in AI-driven healthcare, particularly around data privacy and patient consent. Issues such as ensuring the transparency of AI algorithms used in medical decision-making, maintaining patient confidentiality, and addressing biases in AI models are critical ethical concerns.

AI with Future Directions and Innovation in Healthcare

Company: NVIDIA

Example: NVIDIA is advancing AI in healthcare with platforms like Clara AI, which supports medical imaging analysis, genomic sequencing, and drug discovery. Future innovations may include AI-driven robotic surgeries, virtual health assistants, and further integration of AI into clinical decision support systems to improve patient outcomes.

These examples highlight how AI is being applied across various aspects of healthcare, from diagnostics and treatment planning to operational efficiency and ethical considerations, shaping the future of medicine.

1.1 Historical Evolution and Milestones of AI in Medicine

Artificial Intelligence (AI) has significantly evolved in the field of medicine, marking milestones that have transformed healthcare delivery and patient outcomes.

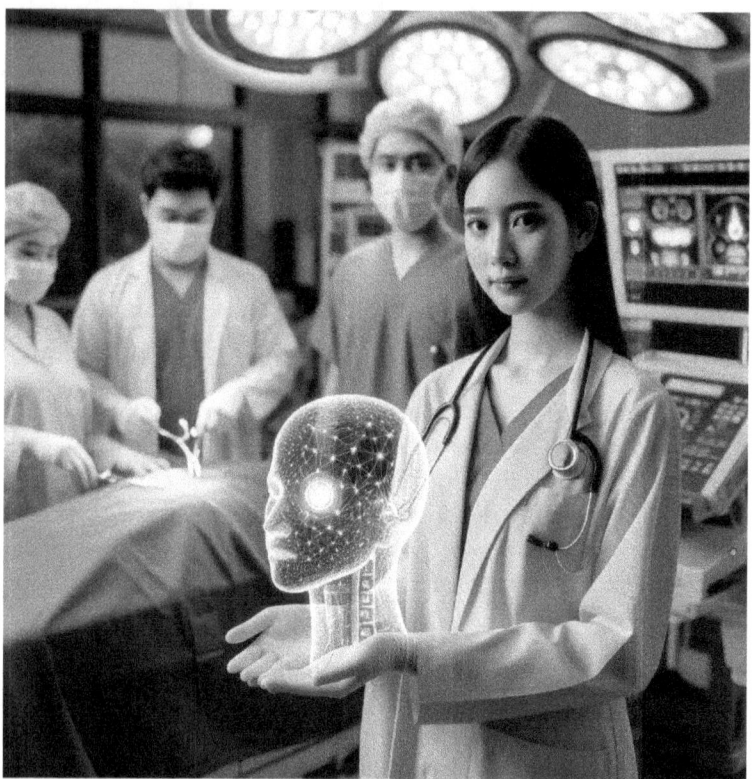

Here's an exploration of the historical evolution and key milestones of AI in medicine:

1. **Early Beginnings and Foundation:** AI in medicine traces its roots to the 1960s, when researchers began exploring applications of AI techniques such as rule-based systems and symbolic reasoning in healthcare. Early efforts focused on developing expert systems to assist with diagnostic decision-making and medical knowledge representation.

2. **Diagnostic Imaging Advancements:** In the 1980s and 1990s, AI made significant strides in diagnostic imaging interpretation. Radiology benefited from AI algorithms capable of analyzing medical images, such as X-rays, CT scans, and MRIs. Computer-aided detection (CAD) systems emerged, assisting radiologists in detecting abnormalities and improving diagnostic accuracy.

3. **Clinical Decision Support Systems (CDSS):** By the late 1990s and early 2000s, AI-powered Clinical Decision Support Systems (CDSS) gained prominence. These systems integrated patient data with medical knowledge databases and AI algorithms to assist clinicians in diagnosis, treatment planning, and medication selection. CDSS improved clinical outcomes by providing evidence-based recommendations and reducing medical errors.

4. **Genomics and Personalized Medicine:** The advancement of AI in genomics has revolutionized personalized medicine. AI algorithms analyze genomic data to predict disease risks, optimize treatment responses based on genetic profiles, and identify potential drug targets. This capability has accelerated the development of targeted therapies and precision medicine approaches.

5. **Natural Language Processing (NLP) and Electronic Health Records (EHR):** AI-driven Natural Language Processing (NLP) capabilities have transformed the utilization of Electronic Health Records (EHR). AI algorithms extract valuable insights from unstructured clinical notes, enabling comprehensive patient data analysis, disease surveillance, and quality improvement initiatives. NLP enhances clinical documentation efficiency and supports population health management.

6. **Surgical Robotics and Minimally Invasive Procedures:** The integration of AI in surgical robotics has enhanced precision, dexterity, and visualization in minimally invasive surgeries. AI-powered robotic systems assist surgeons in performing complex

procedures with greater accuracy and reduced recovery times. Surgical robots have revolutionized specialties such as urology, cardiothoracic surgery, and neurosurgery.

7. **Drug Discovery and Development:** AI accelerates drug discovery by analyzing vast biomedical datasets, predicting drug-target interactions, and optimizing compound synthesis. Machine learning models expedite the identification of potential drug candidates, reducing time and costs associated with traditional drug development processes. AI also aids in repurposing existing drugs for new therapeutic uses.

8. **Telemedicine and Remote Patient Monitoring:** AI technologies support telemedicine initiatives by enabling remote consultations, diagnostics, and continuous patient monitoring. Virtual health assistants equipped with AI algorithms provide personalized care recommendations, detect early signs of deterioration, and improve access to healthcare in remote or underserved areas.

In summary, the historical evolution of AI in medicine has marked significant milestones across various domains, from diagnostic imaging and clinical decision support to personalized medicine and surgical robotics. By leveraging AI technologies, healthcare providers can enhance diagnostic accuracy, optimize treatment outcomes, and improve operational efficiency. Embracing AI-driven innovations continues to redefine healthcare delivery, paving the way for future advancements in medical research, patient care, and population health management.

Examples:

1. **Early Beginnings and Foundation for AI Healthcare during 1960's**

   Example: IBM Watson Health

   Details: IBM has been a pioneer in AI applications for healthcare since the 1960s, developing early systems that laid the foundation for AI in medical diagnostics and data analysis.

2. **Diagnostic Imaging Advancements in Healthcare during 1980s and 1990s**

   Example: GE Healthcare's Centricity Imaging Analytics

   Details: GE Healthcare has been at the forefront of integrating AI into diagnostic imaging systems, enhancing accuracy and efficiency in interpreting medical images such as X-rays, MRIs, and CT scans.

3. **Clinical Decision Support Systems (CDSS) during late 1990s and early 2000s**

   Example: Epic Systems' EpicCare

   Details: EpicCare incorporates AI-driven clinical decision support capabilities, providing healthcare professionals with real-time guidance and data-driven insights to improve patient care and outcomes.

4. **AI in Genomics and Personalized Medicine**

   Example: 23andMe

   Details: 23andMe utilizes AI algorithms to analyze genetic data and provide personalized health insights, predicting disease risks and guiding personalized healthcare decisions based on individual genetic profiles.

5. **AI in Natural Language Processing (NLP) and Electronic Health Records (EHR)**

   Example: Cerner Corporation's HealtheIntent

   Details: Cerner's HealtheIntent platform employs AI-powered NLP to extract meaningful information from unstructured EHR data, enabling better clinical decision-making and population health management.

6. **AI Powered Surgical Robotics and Minimally Invasive Procedures**

   Example: Intuitive Surgical's da Vinci Surgical System

   Details: The da Vinci Surgical System integrates AI to assist surgeons in performing minimally invasive procedures with enhanced precision and dexterity, reducing recovery times and improving surgical outcomes.

7. **AI Powered Drug Discovery and Development**

   Example: Atomwise

   Details: Atomwise uses AI-driven virtual screening to accelerate drug discovery by predicting the binding affinity of small molecules to target proteins, significantly reducing the time and cost involved in identifying potential drug candidates.

8. **AI Powered Telemedicine and Remote Patient Monitoring**

   Example: Teladoc Health

   Details: Teladoc Health utilizes AI for telemedicine consultations and remote patient monitoring, providing real-time health data analysis and virtual care delivery to patients worldwide, improving access to healthcare services.

These examples illustrate how various companies and technologies have leveraged AI to innovate and advance different aspects of healthcare delivery and management over the decades.

1.2 Overview of AI Technologies in Healthcare

Artificial Intelligence (AI) technologies are increasingly pivotal in transforming the healthcare landscape, offering capabilities that enhance patient care, optimize operations, and drive medical innovation.

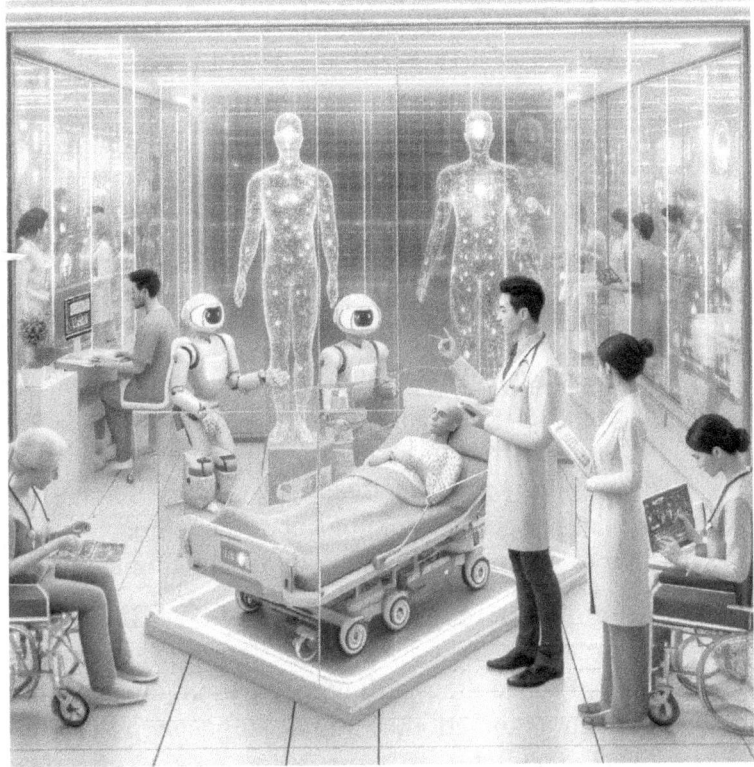

Here are some key reasons why AI adoption is crucial in healthcare:

1. **Enhanced Diagnosis and Treatment:** AI enables more accurate and timely diagnosis by analyzing complex medical data such as imaging scans, genetic information, and patient records. Machine learning algorithms can detect patterns and anomalies that

may indicate diseases or conditions at early stages, leading to proactive treatment interventions.

2. **Clinical Decision Support:** AI-powered systems provide clinicians with decision support tools that integrate patient data, medical research, and clinical guidelines. This assists healthcare providers in making evidence-based decisions about treatment plans, medication choices, and personalized therapies.

3. **Medical Imaging and Analysis:** AI enhances medical imaging interpretation by improving the accuracy of radiology and pathology assessments. Deep learning algorithms can analyze images for abnormalities, tumors, fractures, or other conditions with high precision, aiding in quicker diagnosis and treatment planning.

4. **Personalized Medicine:** AI algorithms analyze large datasets to identify genetic, environmental, and lifestyle factors influencing individual health. This enables personalized treatment plans tailored to a patient's specific biological characteristics and medical history, optimizing therapeutic outcomes.

5. **Administrative Efficiency and Healthcare Operations:** AI streamlines administrative tasks such as scheduling, billing, and patient management through automation. Natural language processing (NLP) facilitates efficient documentation and data entry, reducing administrative burden on healthcare staff.

6. **Drug Discovery and Development:** AI accelerates drug discovery processes by predicting molecular interactions, simulating drug effects, and identifying potential candidates for clinical trials. This enhances the efficiency of pharmaceutical research and

development, bringing new therapies to market faster.

7. **Remote Monitoring and Telemedicine:** AI enables remote monitoring of patients' health metrics in real-time, using wearable devices and IoT sensors. This facilitates proactive healthcare interventions and enables virtual consultations, improving access to healthcare services especially in remote or underserved areas.

8. **Healthcare Fraud Detection and Risk Management:** AI algorithms analyze healthcare data to detect anomalies, identify fraudulent activities, and manage healthcare risks such as patient safety issues or compliance violations. This enhances overall healthcare system integrity and patient safety.

In summary, the adoption of AI technologies in healthcare is essential for advancing patient care, improving clinical outcomes, and optimizing healthcare delivery. By leveraging AI for diagnosis, treatment planning, personalized medicine, and operational efficiency, healthcare organizations can enhance medical practices, mitigate risks, and ultimately improve the quality of life for patients worldwide.

Examples:

1. **Enhanced Diagnosis and Treatment**

   > **Example:** IBM Watson Health
   >
   > **Details:** IBM Watson Health utilizes AI to assist healthcare providers in diagnosing and treating complex medical conditions by analyzing vast amounts of patient data, medical literature, and clinical guidelines to provide evidence-based recommendations.

2. **Clinical Decision Support**

> **Example:** Cerner Corporation's HealtheIntent
>
> **Details:** Cerner's HealtheIntent platform incorporates AI-driven clinical decision support capabilities to aid healthcare professionals in making informed decisions at the point of care, improving clinical outcomes and patient safety.

3. **Medical Imaging and Analysis**

> **Example:** Siemens Healthineers' AI-Rad Companion
>
> **Details:** AI-Rad Companion by Siemens Healthineers uses AI algorithms to assist radiologists in interpreting medical imaging scans such as MRIs, CT scans, and X-rays, providing faster and more accurate diagnostics.

4. **Personalized Medicine**

> **Example:** Foundation Medicine
>
> **Details:** Foundation Medicine applies AI to genomic data analysis to deliver personalized cancer treatment options based on the molecular profile of each patient's tumor, enhancing treatment efficacy and patient outcomes.

5. **Administrative Efficiency and Healthcare Operations**

> **Example:** Epic Systems' EpicCare
>
> **Details:** EpicCare includes AI-driven administrative tools that optimize healthcare operations by streamlining scheduling, billing, and resource allocation, improving efficiency within healthcare organizations.

6. **Drug Discovery and Development**

> **Example:** Atomwise
>
> **Details:** Atomwise employs AI-driven virtual screening to accelerate drug discovery by predicting the binding affinity of small molecules to target proteins, enabling faster identification of potential drug candidates for various diseases.

7. **Remote Monitoring and Telemedicine**

> **Example:** Teladoc Health

Details: Teladoc Health utilizes AI for remote patient monitoring and telemedicine consultations, enabling real-time health data analysis and virtual care delivery, particularly valuable in remote or underserved areas.

8. **Healthcare Fraud Detection and Risk Management**

Example: Optum Fraud and Abuse Detection System

Details: Optum's system uses AI algorithms to analyze healthcare claims data and detect patterns indicative of fraud, waste, or abuse, helping payers and providers mitigate financial risks and ensure compliance with regulatory standards.

These examples demonstrate how AI is integrated into various aspects of healthcare to improve diagnosis, treatment, operational efficiency, and patient outcomes while addressing specific challenges such as personalized medicine and fraud detection.

2. AI in Medical Imaging and Diagnostics

Artificial Intelligence (AI) is revolutionizing medical imaging and diagnostics, offering transformative capabilities that enhance healthcare delivery, diagnosis accuracy, and patient outcomes.

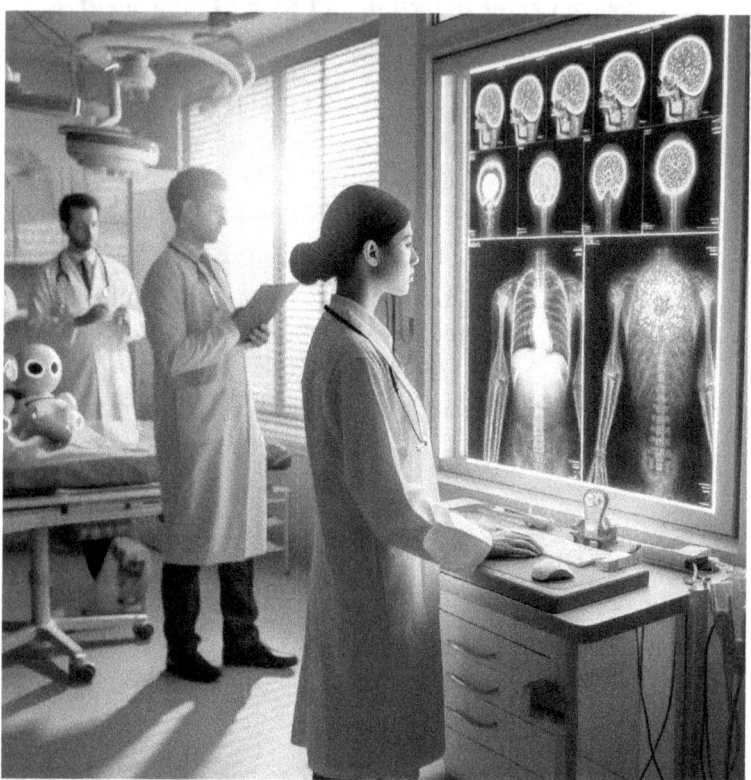

Here's a comprehensive exploration of why AI adoption in medical imaging and diagnostics is crucial:

1. **AI for Enhanced Diagnostic Accuracy and Speed:** AI-powered algorithms analyze medical images such as X-rays, CT scans, MRI scans, and pathology slides with precision and speed. By detecting subtle patterns and anomalies that may not be visible to the human eye, AI enhances diagnostic accuracy. This capability supports radiologists and pathologists in making more informed

decisions, leading to early detection of diseases, accurate diagnoses, and timely interventions.

2. **Automation of Image Analysis and Workflow Optimization:** AI automates the analysis of medical images, reducing the time-consuming task of manual interpretation. Machine learning models can segment organs, identify lesions, measure tumor growth, and quantify tissue characteristics, streamlining radiology and pathology workflows. Automation improves operational efficiency, accelerates reporting turnaround times, and enhances overall healthcare productivity.

3. **Personalized Treatment Planning and Precision Medicine:** AI facilitates personalized treatment planning by integrating imaging data with clinical and genomic information. Machine learning algorithms predict treatment responses, stratify patient populations based on imaging biomarkers, and tailor therapies to individual patient profiles. This personalized approach optimizes treatment outcomes, minimizes adverse effects, and advances precision medicine initiatives across specialties.

4. **Innovation in Imaging Technology and Research:** AI drives innovation in imaging technology by enhancing the capabilities of medical devices and modalities. AI algorithms improve image quality, reduce noise, and enhance resolution, leading to clearer diagnostic images. Additionally, AI supports medical research by analyzing large-scale imaging datasets, identifying disease patterns, and facilitating the development of new diagnostic techniques and therapies.

5. **Integration with Clinical Decision Support Systems (CDSS):** AI-powered Clinical Decision Support Systems integrate imaging data with patient records and medical knowledge databases. These systems provide real-time diagnostic assistance, suggest relevant clinical guidelines, and alert healthcare providers to critical findings. AI-driven CDSS enhances diagnostic confidence, reduces

diagnostic errors, and supports evidence-based decision-making in clinical practice.

6. **Ethical Considerations and Regulatory Compliance:** The adoption of AI in medical imaging raises ethical considerations related to patient privacy, data security, and algorithmic transparency. Ensuring ethical AI deployment involves safeguarding patient confidentiality, mitigating biases in AI algorithms, and adhering to regulatory guidelines. Transparent AI systems foster trust among healthcare professionals and patients, ensuring responsible use of AI technologies in medical imaging and diagnostics.

7. **Cost Efficiency and Resource Optimization:** AI in medical imaging optimizes resource allocation by improving the efficiency of diagnostic processes and reducing healthcare costs. Automated image analysis reduces the need for repetitive tasks and enhances workflow efficiency, allowing healthcare facilities to handle larger patient volumes without compromising quality of care. Cost savings from AI adoption can be redirected to enhancing patient care and investing in advanced medical technologies.

8. **Future Directions and Clinical Adoption:** AI continues to evolve in medical imaging with ongoing advancements in deep learning, computer vision, and image recognition technologies. Future developments aim to enhance AI interpretability, integrate multimodal imaging data, and expand AI applications across diverse clinical specialties. Clinical adoption of AI-driven imaging solutions is pivotal in realizing the full potential of AI to improve healthcare delivery and patient outcomes globally.

In summary, the integration of AI in medical imaging and diagnostics is pivotal for enhancing diagnostic accuracy, optimizing workflows, and advancing personalized medicine. By harnessing AI technologies, healthcare providers can deliver timely and precise diagnoses, improve patient care quality, and drive innovation in medical imaging practices. Embracing AI enables healthcare organizations to navigate complex healthcare challenges, achieve operational excellence, and pave the way for transformative advancements in healthcare delivery.

Examples:

1. **Enhanced Diagnostic Accuracy and Speed**

Company: Aidoc
Example: Aidoc uses AI algorithms to enhance diagnostic accuracy and speed in radiology by analyzing medical imaging scans (such as CT and MRI). Their AI-powered platform assists radiologists in detecting abnormalities like intracranial hemorrhages and pulmonary embolisms with greater efficiency and accuracy.

2. **Automation of Image Analysis and Workflow Optimization**

Company: Arterys
Example: Arterys provides AI-powered solutions for medical imaging analysis, particularly in cardiology and oncology. Their platform automates image interpretation tasks like tumor measurements and cardiac function assessments, optimizing workflow efficiency for healthcare providers.

3. **Personalized Treatment Planning and Precision Medicine**

Company: Tempus
Example: Tempus leverages AI and machine learning to analyze clinical and molecular data from cancer patients. Their platform helps oncologists personalize treatment plans based on individual genetic profiles, improving outcomes through precision medicine approaches.

4. **Innovation in Imaging Technology and Research**

Company: Butterfly Network

> **Example:** Butterfly Network develops handheld ultrasound devices combined with AI algorithms. Their technology enables healthcare professionals to perform high-quality imaging at the point of care, enhancing diagnostic capabilities and expanding access to imaging technology globally.

5. **Integration with Clinical Decision Support Systems (CDSS)**

> **Company: IBM Watson Health**
>
> **Example:** IBM Watson Health integrates AI into clinical decision support systems within electronic health records (EHR). Their AI-powered tools analyze patient data, medical literature, and treatment guidelines to assist healthcare providers in making evidence-based decisions and improving patient outcomes.

6. **Ethical Considerations and Regulatory Compliance**

> **Company: Google Health**
>
> **Example:** Google Health addresses ethical considerations and regulatory compliance in AI-driven healthcare solutions. They focus on ensuring patient privacy, transparency in AI algorithms, and compliance with healthcare regulations such as GDPR and HIPAA to maintain trust and ethical standards.

7. **Cost Efficiency and Resource Optimization**

> Company: Olive
>
> Example: Olive AI provides solutions for automating administrative and operational tasks in healthcare facilities. Their AI-driven platform optimizes resource allocation, reduces administrative costs, and enhances efficiency in areas such as revenue cycle management and supply chain logistics.

8. **Future Directions and Clinical Adoption**

> **Example:** Philips Healthcare's IntelliSpace AI Workflow Suite
>
> **Details:** Philips Healthcare integrates AI image analytics into its IntelliSpace AI Workflow Suite to assist radiologists and clinicians in interpreting medical images more accurately and efficiently. The platform leverages AI algorithms to analyze imaging data and provide insights that support clinical decision-making, improving diagnostic accuracy and patient care outcomes.

9. **Integration Image Analytics with Clinical Decision Support Systems (CDSS)**

> **Example:** GE Healthcare's Centricity Imaging Analytics
>
> **Details:** GE Healthcare's Centricity Imaging Analytics integrates AI image analytics with clinical decision support systems to enhance diagnostic capabilities across various medical specialties. The system uses AI algorithms to analyze and interpret medical images, providing clinicians with actionable insights and recommendations that align with evidence-based guidelines, thereby improving patient care and workflow efficiency.

These examples demonstrate how AI technologies are transforming healthcare by improving diagnostic capabilities, optimizing workflows, enabling personalized medicine, advancing imaging technology, integrating with clinical decision support, addressing ethical concerns, and optimizing resource utilization. As AI continues to evolve, its impact on healthcare is expected to further enhance patient care and operational efficiency across the industry.

2.1 AI Algorithms for Image Analysis and Interpretation

Artificial Intelligence (AI) algorithms are revolutionizing image analysis and interpretation across various industries, including healthcare, manufacturing, and autonomous systems.

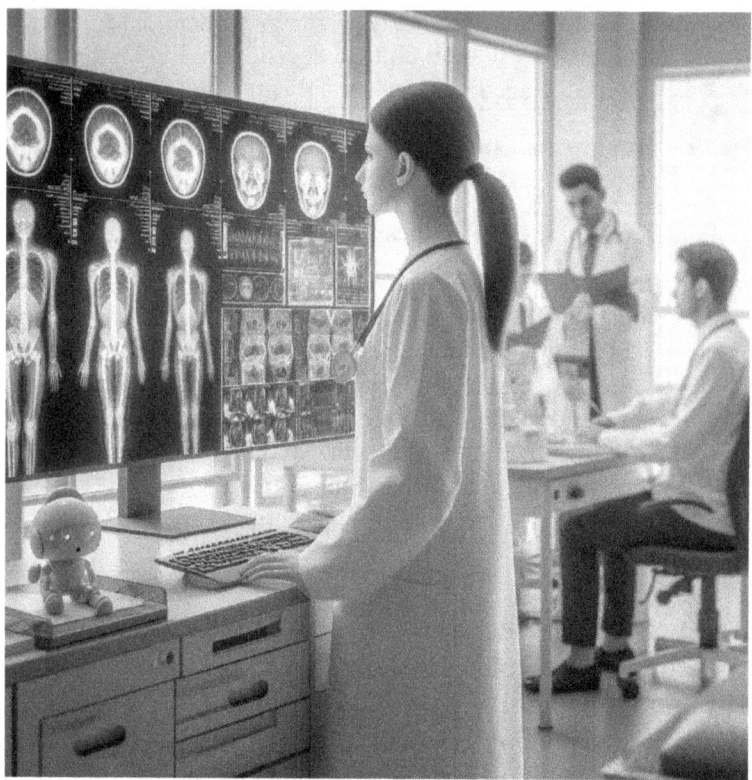

Here's a detailed exploration of why AI adoption in image analysis and interpretation is crucial:

1. **Enhanced Image Recognition and Classification:** AI algorithms excel in image recognition tasks by accurately identifying objects, patterns, and anomalies within images. Deep learning models, such as convolutional neural networks (CNNs), analyze pixel data to classify images based on predefined categories. This capability is pivotal in medical diagnostics for detecting deceases.

2. **Automation of Complex Image Processing Tasks:** AI-powered algorithms automate complex image processing tasks that traditionally require human expertise and time-intensive manual effort. These algorithms can segment images to distinguish regions of interest, extract meaningful features, and enhance image quality by reducing noise and artifacts. Automation in image processing accelerates workflows, improves efficiency, and enables scalable deployment across diverse healthcare applications.

3. **Medical Imaging and Diagnostics Advancements:** In healthcare, AI algorithms enhance medical imaging and diagnostics by interpreting radiological scans (e.g., X-rays, CT scans, MRI) and pathology slides with high accuracy. Machine learning algorithms analyze images to detect abnormalities, quantify disease progression, and assist radiologists and pathologists in making informed diagnostic decisions. AI-driven diagnostics improve patient outcomes by enabling early detection of diseases and facilitating personalized treatment planning.

4. **Facilitation of Medical Research:** AI algorithms enable large-scale analysis of medical imaging data across diverse patient populations. This capability aids researchers in identifying trends, correlations, and potential new biomarkers, accelerating medical discoveries and advancements in treatment protocols.

5. **Predictive Analytics for Proactive Healthcare:** Leveraging historical imaging data, AI algorithms can predict disease progression, assess treatment response, and anticipate patient outcomes. This predictive analytics capability supports proactive healthcare management and enables timely interventions to improve patient prognosis.

6. **Enhanced Operational Efficiency:** AI-driven automation of routine tasks such as image preprocessing, segmentation, and feature extraction enhances operational efficiency within radiology and pathology departments.

This efficiency gains allow healthcare providers to focus more on complex cases and patient interaction.

7. **Cost Efficiency and Resource Optimization:** By reducing diagnostic errors, optimizing workflow, and improving treatment efficacy, AI algorithms contribute to cost savings in healthcare delivery. They help minimize unnecessary tests, shorten hospital stays, and allocate resources more effectively, thereby lowering overall healthcare expenditures.

8. **Regulatory Compliance and Risk Management:** AI algorithms assist healthcare providers in adhering to regulatory standards and guidelines by ensuring accurate image interpretation and reporting. They also aid in detecting anomalies or deviations that may indicate potential risks, enhancing patient safety and healthcare quality.

9. **Integration with Clinical Decision Support Systems:** AI algorithms can be integrated into clinical decision support systems (CDSS) to provide real-time insights and recommendations based on imaging data. This integration supports healthcare professionals in making evidence-based decisions, improving patient care quality and safety.

10. **Remote and Telemedicine Capabilities:** AI-powered image analysis enables remote interpretation of medical images, facilitating telemedicine consultations and collaborations between healthcare providers across different locations. This capability enhances access to specialized care, particularly in rural or underserved areas.

11. **Facilitation of Surgical Planning and Guidance:** Advanced AI algorithms assist surgeons in preoperative planning by analyzing complex anatomical structures from imaging data. During surgery, AI can provide real-time guidance, improving precision and reducing procedural risks.

12. **Continuous Learning and Improvement:** AI algorithms can be trained using vast amounts of annotated imaging data to continuously learn and improve their accuracy and reliability over time. This iterative learning process enhances algorithm performance and ensures adaptation to evolving medical knowledge and practices.

13. **Detection of Rare and Complex Conditions:** AI algorithms excel in identifying rare diseases or complex conditions that may present unique challenges in diagnosis and treatment planning. Their ability to analyze patterns across diverse cases enhances diagnostic capabilities and expands clinical insights.

14. **Support for Population Health Management:** By analyzing population-level imaging data, AI algorithms contribute to population health management initiatives. They help identify health trends, assess disease prevalence, and prioritize public health interventions, thereby promoting preventive healthcare strategies.

15. **Enhanced Patient Engagement and Education:** AI-powered imaging solutions can generate visual reports and educational materials based on imaging findings, enhancing patient understanding of their conditions and treatment options. This engagement fosters informed decision-making and improves patient compliance.

16. **Ethical Considerations and Bias Mitigation:** The adoption of AI in image analysis necessitates ethical considerations, including transparency, fairness, and bias mitigation. AI algorithms must be trained on diverse datasets to minimize biases in image interpretation, ensuring equitable outcomes across demographics and geographic regions. Transparent AI systems enhance trust among stakeholders and promote responsible deployment in sensitive domains such as healthcare and criminal justice.

17. **Future Directions and Innovation in AI Image Analysis:** AI continues to evolve in image analysis with advancements in deep learning architectures, multimodal

data integration, and explainable AI models. Future developments aim to enhance AI interpretability, integrate contextual information from multiple sources, and expand AI applications in emerging fields such as augmented reality and autonomous navigation systems. Continued research and development in AI algorithms for image analysis promise to unlock new possibilities in innovation and societal impact.

In summary, the adoption of AI algorithms for image analysis and interpretation in healthcare is essential for improving diagnostic accuracy, enhancing personalized patient care, facilitating medical research, and optimizing operational efficiency. By leveraging AI technologies, healthcare organizations can achieve better patient outcomes, reduce costs, and drive innovation in medical imaging and diagnostics.

Examples:

1. **Enhanced Image Recognition and Classification:**

   Company: Aidoc

   Example: Aidoc uses AI to analyze medical images such as CT scans and MRIs to detect abnormalities like intracranial hemorrhages or pulmonary embolisms with high accuracy, helping radiologists prioritize urgent cases.

2. **Automation of Complex Image Processing Tasks:**

   Company: Zebra Medical Vision

   Example: Zebra Medical Vision automates the analysis of medical imaging data using AI algorithms to assist radiologists in detecting various conditions, including osteoporosis and cardiovascular diseases, enhancing diagnostic efficiency.

3. **Medical Imaging and Diagnostics Advancements:**

   Company: GE Healthcare

   Example: GE Healthcare incorporates AI into its medical imaging devices and software solutions to improve image quality, accelerate image interpretation, and provide insights for more precise diagnostics across various modalities like ultrasound, MRI, and X-ray.

4. **Facilitation of Medical Research:**

   Company: PathAI

   Example: PathAI utilizes AI algorithms to analyze pathology images, aiding researchers in identifying biomarkers, predicting treatment responses, and advancing discoveries in oncology and other fields through large-scale image data analysis.

5. **Predictive Analytics for Proactive Healthcare:**

   Company: Gauss Surgical

   Example: Gauss Surgical's AI platform uses computer vision to estimate blood loss during surgeries based on real-time analysis of images from surgical sponges, enabling proactive management of patient care and reducing complications.

6. **Enhanced Operational Efficiency:**

   Company: Arterys

   Example: Arterys employs AI for cloud-based medical imaging analytics, allowing clinicians to analyze and share medical images efficiently. This technology enhances workflow productivity and collaboration among healthcare professionals.

7. **Cost Efficiency and Resource Optimization:**

   Company: Nuance Communications

   Example: Nuance provides AI-powered solutions for medical imaging documentation and workflow optimization. Their technology reduces transcription costs, enhances report turnaround times, and improves resource allocation in radiology departments.

8. **Regulatory Compliance and Risk Management:**

   Company: Blackford Analysis

Example: Blackford Analysis offers AI-powered software that standardizes image processing workflows while ensuring compliance with regulatory standards and protocols, enhancing quality control and patient safety in medical imaging.

9. **Integration with Clinical Decision Support Systems:**

Company: Enlitic

Example: Enlitic integrates AI into clinical decision support systems to assist radiologists in interpreting medical images more accurately and efficiently. Their technology helps in diagnosing diseases like lung cancer and fractures with improved precision.

10. **Remote and Telemedicine Capabilities:**

Company: Aidoc (again)

Example: Aidoc's AI-powered platform supports telemedicine by providing remote radiology services. Their technology enables healthcare providers to review and diagnose medical images from different locations, improving access to specialized care.

11. **Facilitation of Surgical Planning and Guidance:**

Company: Stryker

Example: Stryker utilizes AI-enhanced imaging technologies for surgical planning and navigation. Their systems integrate AI algorithms to assist surgeons in visualizing patient anatomy and performing procedures with greater precision and safety.

12. **Continuous Learning and Improvement:**

Company: Quibim

Example: Quibim applies AI to continuously analyze and learn from medical imaging data, supporting ongoing improvements in diagnostic accuracy and treatment planning across various medical specialties.

13. **Detection of Rare and Complex Conditions:**

> **Company: Viz.ai**
>
> **Example:** Viz.ai specializes in using AI to analyze medical imaging for the early detection of stroke. Their technology automatically alerts neurovascular specialists to cases of suspected large vessel occlusion, enabling timely interventions and improving patient outcomes.

14. **Support for Population Health:**

> **Company: Philips Healthcare**
>
> **Example:** Philips Healthcare employs AI to analyze population-level imaging data for insights into disease prevalence and healthcare trends. Their solutions help healthcare organizations optimize resource allocation and public health interventions.

15. **Enhanced Patient Engagement and Education:**

> **Company: Proximie**
>
> **Example:** Proximie utilizes AI-powered augmented reality (AR) technology to enhance patient engagement during medical imaging procedures. Their platform allows clinicians to interact with patients in real-time, explaining imaging results and treatment options visually.

16. **Ethical Considerations and Bias Mitigation:**

> **Company: Google Health**
>
> **Example:** Google Health addresses ethical considerations in AI-driven healthcare by developing rigorous guidelines for data privacy, algorithm transparency, and bias mitigation in medical imaging analytics, ensuring fair and equitable patient care.

17. **Future Directions and Innovation :**

> **Company: NVIDIA**
>
> **Example:** NVIDIA continues to innovate in AI image analysis for healthcare by developing advanced GPU-based

> platforms that accelerate AI algorithms in medical imaging. Their technology supports future applications in real-time diagnostics, personalized medicine, and AI-driven healthcare research.

These examples showcase how various companies are leveraging AI image analytics to transform healthcare delivery, improve patient outcomes, and advance medical research while addressing ethical considerations and driving innovation in the field.

2.2 Applications of AI in Radiology and Pathology

Artificial Intelligence (AI) is revolutionizing the fields of radiology and pathology by enhancing diagnostic accuracy, optimizing workflow efficiency, and improving patient outcomes.

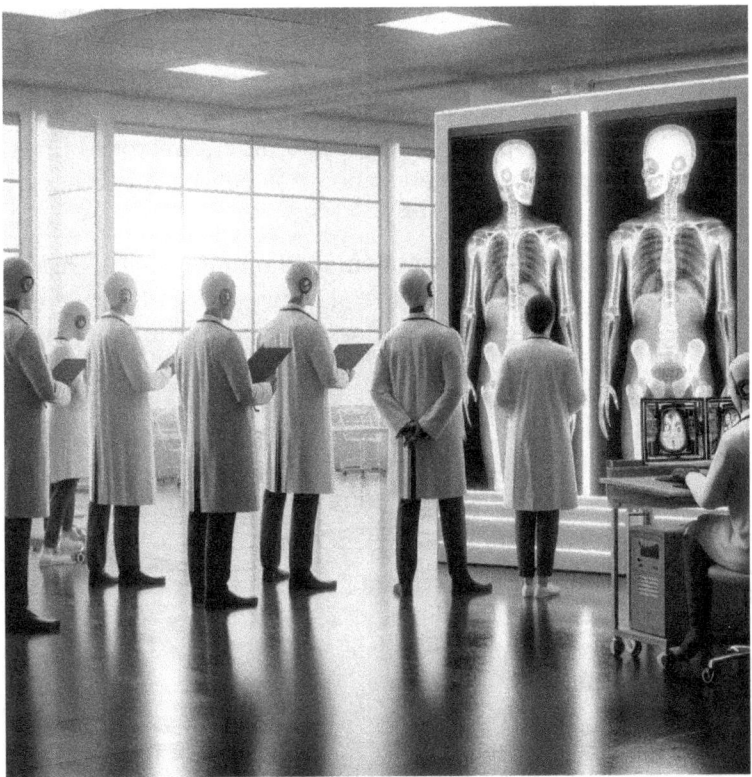

Here's an in-depth exploration of why AI adoption in radiology and pathology is crucial:

1. **Enhanced Diagnostic Accuracy in radiology and pathology:** AI algorithms in radiology and pathology enable more accurate and timely diagnosis by analyzing medical images and pathology slides with high precision. Machine learning models, such as convolutional neural networks (CNNs), can detect subtle anomalies, classify diseases, and assist radiologists and pathologists in

interpreting complex data. This capability significantly reduces diagnostic errors and enhances clinical decision-making.

2. **Workflow Optimization and Efficiency:** AI-powered tools streamline radiology and pathology workflows by automating routine tasks, such as image analysis, annotation, and report generation. AI algorithms analyze large volumes of medical images and pathology specimens efficiently, allowing healthcare professionals to focus on critical tasks and expedite diagnosis. Workflow optimization leads to faster turnaround times, improved resource allocation, and enhanced patient care delivery.

3. **Personalized Treatment Planning:** AI enables personalized treatment planning in radiology and pathology by integrating patient-specific data with medical imaging and pathology findings. AI algorithms analyze imaging biomarkers, genetic information, and clinical data to tailor treatment strategies based on individual patient profiles. Personalized approaches optimize therapeutic outcomes, minimize treatment-related risks, and improve overall patient management.

4. **Research and Development Advancements:** AI fosters innovation in radiology and pathology research by facilitating large-scale data analysis, pattern recognition, and predictive modeling. AI-driven research identifies new biomarkers, correlates imaging features with disease progression, and explores novel therapeutic targets. These insights accelerate medical discoveries, support evidence-based medicine, and drive advancements in diagnostic techniques and treatment protocols.

5. **Quality Assurance and Standardization:** AI algorithms ensure quality assurance and standardization in radiology and pathology practices by automating quality control processes and adhering to clinical guidelines. AI-driven quality assurance tools detect imaging artifacts, validate diagnostic protocols, and ensure consistency in

pathological assessments. Standardized practices enhance diagnostic reliability, reduce variability in interpretations, and promote healthcare accreditation compliance.

6. **Telemedicine and Remote Diagnosis:** AI facilitates telemedicine initiatives in radiology and pathology by enabling remote image interpretation and consultation. AI-powered telemedicine platforms securely transmit medical images and pathology slides to specialists worldwide for timely diagnosis and treatment recommendations. Telemedicine capabilities enhance healthcare access, particularly in underserved regions, and support collaborative decision-making among healthcare teams.

7. **Ethical Considerations and Regulatory Compliance:** The adoption of AI in radiology and pathology necessitates ethical considerations, including patient privacy protection, transparency in AI algorithms, and regulatory compliance with healthcare standards. AI systems must adhere to ethical guidelines, ensure data security, and mitigate biases in medical image analysis and pathology interpretations. Ethical practices uphold patient trust, uphold confidentiality, and safeguard sensitive healthcare information.

8. **Future Directions and Innovation in AI Applications:** The future of AI in radiology and pathology holds promise for advancing imaging technologies, integrating multimodal data sources, and enhancing clinical decision support systems. Ongoing research aims to develop explainable AI models, expand AI applications in oncology and neurology, and integrate AI with emerging imaging modalities. Continued innovation in AI-driven diagnostics promises to redefine healthcare delivery, improve diagnostic accuracy, and optimize patient outcomes.

In summary, AI applications in radiology and pathology are pivotal in transforming healthcare delivery, improving diagnostic capabilities, and advancing medical research. By leveraging AI technologies, healthcare institutions can achieve higher diagnostic accuracy, optimize operational efficiency, and deliver personalized patient care. Embracing AI-driven innovations enables healthcare providers to meet evolving clinical challenges, enhance healthcare outcomes, and pave the way for a more efficient and equitable healthcare system.

Examples:

1. **Enhanced Diagnostic Accuracy:**

   Company: Aidoc

   Example: Aidoc's AI algorithms analyze radiology images such as CT scans and MRIs to assist radiologists in detecting critical findings like intracranial hemorrhages and pulmonary embolisms with high accuracy, improving diagnostic speed and accuracy.

2. **Workflow Optimization and Efficiency:**

   Company: Zebra Medical Vision

   Example: Zebra Medical Vision automates the analysis of medical imaging data using AI algorithms to prioritize and triage radiology exams. Their technology helps in optimizing radiologists' workflow by flagging urgent cases and reducing turnaround times for routine exams.

3. **Personalized Treatment Planning:**

   Company: PathAI

   Example: PathAI utilizes AI to analyze pathology images and identify biomarkers that can personalize treatment plans for cancer patients. Their platform supports oncologists in making informed decisions based on precise diagnostic insights derived from image data.

4. **Research and Development Advancements:**

   Company: Google Health

   Example: Google Health applies AI to medical imaging research by developing algorithms that analyze vast amounts of imaging data to identify patterns and correlations in diseases. Their research aims to advance diagnostic capabilities and treatment outcomes across various medical specialties.

5. **Quality Assurance and Standardization:**

   Company: Proscia

   Example: Proscia's AI-driven platform standardizes and automates pathology image analysis, ensuring consistency and accuracy in diagnostic procedures. Their technology helps pathology labs maintain high-quality standards and reduce variability in diagnoses.

6. **Telemedicine and Remote Diagnosis:**

   Company: InferVision

   Example: InferVision develops AI solutions for telemedicine, enabling remote diagnosis and consultation through automated analysis of medical images such as chest X-rays. Their technology facilitates access to expert opinions and reduces geographical barriers to healthcare.

7. **Ethical Considerations and Regulatory Compliance:**

   Company: Arterys

   Example: Arterys addresses ethical considerations by ensuring transparency and compliance with regulatory standards in AI-driven medical imaging analytics. Their platform emphasizes patient privacy protection and algorithmic transparency to maintain trust and ethical standards.

8. **Future Directions and Innovation in AI Applications:**

   Company: NVIDIA

   Example: NVIDIA continues to innovate in AI applications for medical imaging by developing GPU-based platforms that accelerate AI algorithms in radiology and pathology. Their technology supports future

> advancements in real-time diagnostics, personalized medicine, and AI-driven healthcare research.

These examples demonstrate how various companies are leveraging AI algorithms to enhance diagnostic accuracy, optimize workflows, personalize treatment planning, advance research and development, ensure quality assurance, enable telemedicine, address ethical considerations, and drive future innovations in medical imaging analytics in radiology and pathology.

2.3 Enhancing Diagnostic Accuracy with Machine Learning

Machine Learning (ML) is revolutionizing diagnostic processes across various industries, particularly in healthcare, by significantly enhancing accuracy, efficiency, and overall quality of diagnoses.

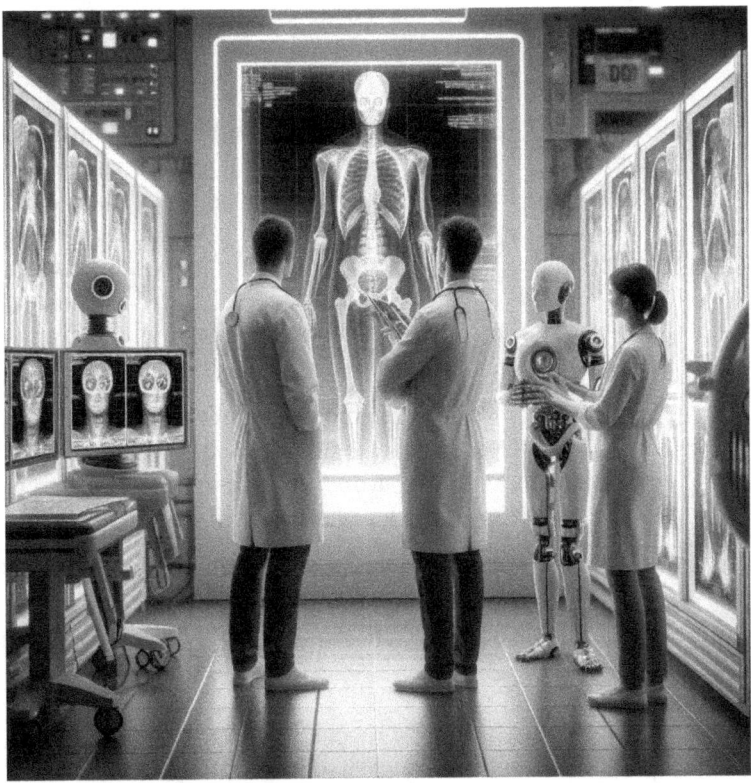

Here's an in-depth exploration of why adopting machine learning for enhancing diagnostic accuracy is crucial:

1. **Improved Decision-making:** Machine learning algorithms analyze vast amounts of patient data, including medical records, imaging studies, and genetic information, to aid healthcare professionals in making more accurate and data-driven diagnostic decisions. By identifying subtle patterns and correlations within

complex datasets, ML enhances diagnostic precision and reduces the likelihood of misdiagnosis.

2. **Automation of Diagnostic Processes:** ML-powered automation streamlines diagnostic workflows by automating routine tasks such as image analysis, pattern recognition, and data interpretation. This automation reduces human error, standardizes diagnostic procedures, and accelerates the diagnostic timeline, leading to faster patient outcomes and improved operational efficiency in healthcare settings.

3. **Enhanced Image Analysis:** In medical imaging, ML algorithms excel in interpreting radiological images (e.g., X-rays, MRI scans, CT scans) and pathology slides with high accuracy. These algorithms can detect anomalies, quantify disease progression, and differentiate between benign and malignant conditions, thereby supporting radiologists and pathologists in making more informed diagnostic assessments.

4. **Personalized Medicine and Treatment Planning:** ML facilitates personalized medicine by integrating patient-specific data with diagnostic findings to tailor treatment plans based on individual health profiles. By analyzing genetic markers, clinical histories, and treatment responses, ML algorithms predict optimal treatment strategies, optimize therapeutic outcomes, and minimize adverse effects, thereby improving patient care and prognosis.

5. **Predictive Analytics for Early Detection:** ML enables predictive analytics by analyzing historical patient data to forecast disease risks, anticipate disease progression, and identify potential complications. Early detection through predictive modeling allows healthcare providers to initiate preventive measures, offer timely interventions, and improve patient outcomes through proactive healthcare management.

6. **Competitive Advantage in Healthcare Delivery:** Healthcare providers leveraging ML for diagnostic

accuracy gain a competitive edge by enhancing clinical capabilities, attracting more patients seeking advanced diagnostic technologies, and positioning themselves as leaders in healthcare innovation. ML-driven diagnostic excellence not only improves patient satisfaction but also strengthens institutional reputation and market competitiveness.

7. **Operational Efficiency and Cost Savings:** ML-driven diagnostic solutions enhance operational efficiency by reducing diagnostic turnaround times, optimizing resource utilization, and minimizing unnecessary procedures or tests. By automating labor-intensive tasks and improving workflow efficiencies, healthcare institutions achieve cost savings, enhance productivity among medical staff, and allocate resources more effectively.

8. **Ethical Considerations and Regulatory Compliance:** The adoption of ML in diagnostic practices necessitates adherence to ethical guidelines, patient confidentiality protections, and regulatory compliance with healthcare standards. Ensuring transparency in ML algorithms, safeguarding patient data privacy, and mitigating biases in diagnostic models are critical to maintaining trust, ethical integrity, and regulatory compliance within healthcare settings.

In summary, the integration of machine learning to enhance diagnostic accuracy represents a transformative shift in healthcare delivery, offering unparalleled opportunities to improve patient outcomes, drive clinical efficiencies, and foster innovation in medical diagnostics. By harnessing the power of ML algorithms, healthcare providers can achieve diagnostic excellence, deliver personalized patient care, and navigate the evolving landscape of modern healthcare with confidence and competence.

Examples:
1. **Improved Decision-making:**

   Company: Qure.ai

Example: Qure.ai uses machine learning algorithms to analyze medical images such as X-rays and CT scans. Their AI-powered platform assists radiologists in making faster and more accurate diagnostic decisions, especially in detecting abnormalities like fractures or brain bleeds.

2. **Automation of Diagnostic Processes:**

Company: Aidoc

Example: Aidoc automates diagnostic processes in radiology by using AI algorithms to flag critical findings in medical imaging exams. Their technology improves workflow efficiency by prioritizing urgent cases and reducing turnaround times for radiology reports.

3. **Enhanced Image Analysis:**

Company: Arterys

Example: Arterys employs machine learning for advanced image analysis in medical imaging. Their AI-powered solutions provide quantitative measurements and 3D visualizations of cardiac MRI and CT scans, aiding cardiologists in precise diagnosis and treatment planning.

4. **Personalized Medicine and Treatment Planning:**

Company: Paige

Example: Paige leverages AI to assist pathologists in personalized medicine by analyzing pathology images. Their platform uses machine learning to identify molecular and cellular patterns, guiding oncologists in tailoring treatment strategies based on individual patient profiles.

5. **Predictive Analytics for Early Detection:**

Company: Zebra Medical Vision

Example: Zebra Medical Vision develops AI algorithms for predictive analytics in medical imaging. Their technology analyzes longitudinal imaging data to detect early signs of diseases such as osteoporosis and breast cancer, enabling proactive healthcare interventions.

6. **Competitive Advantage in Healthcare Delivery:**

> **Company: GE Healthcare**
>
> **Example:** GE Healthcare integrates machine learning into its medical imaging devices and software solutions. Their AI-driven platforms enhance diagnostic accuracy, streamline workflow, and improve patient outcomes, providing healthcare providers with a competitive edge in delivering quality care.

7. **Operational Efficiency and Cost Savings:**

> **Company: Nuance Communications**
>
> **Example:** Nuance Communications offers AI-powered solutions for medical imaging documentation and workflow optimization. Their technology automates reporting processes, reduces transcription costs, and enhances operational efficiency in radiology departments.

8. **Ethical Considerations and Regulatory Compliance:**

> **Company: PathAI (again)**
>
> **Example:** PathAI addresses ethical considerations in AI-driven medical imaging by ensuring transparency and adherence to regulatory standards. Their platform emphasizes data privacy protection and algorithmic validation to maintain ethical integrity and regulatory compliance in pathology analysis.

These examples illustrate how various companies are leveraging machine learning and AI technologies to enhance decision-making, automate diagnostics, improve image analysis, personalize medicine, enable early detection, gain competitive advantages, achieve operational efficiencies, and uphold ethical standards in medical imaging and diagnostics.

3. AI in Predictive Analytics and Disease Prevention

Artificial Intelligence (AI) is reshaping the landscape of healthcare and disease prevention through predictive analytics, offering transformative capabilities that enhance decision-making, improve patient outcomes, and optimize healthcare delivery.

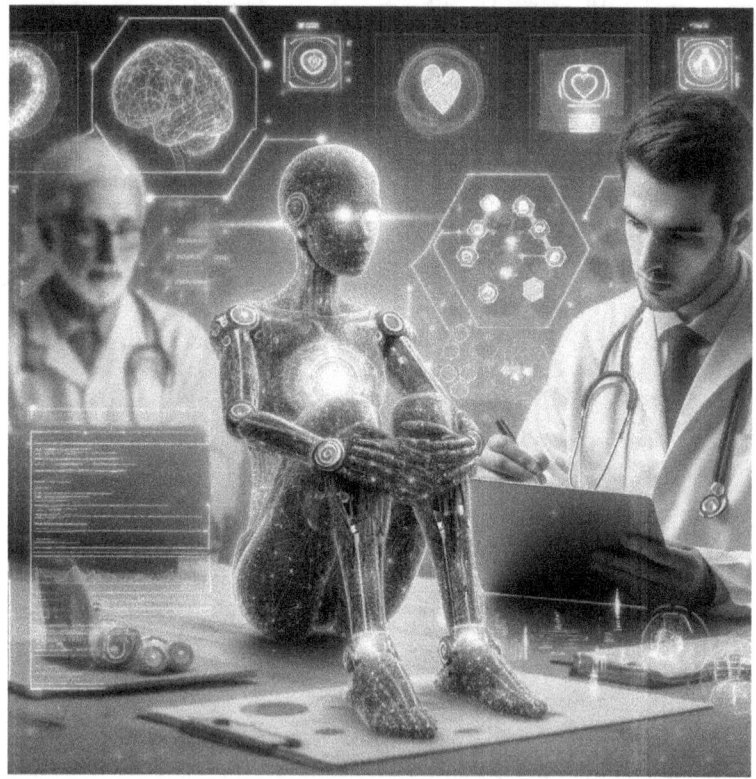

Here's a structured exploration of why AI adoption in predictive analytics and disease prevention is crucial:

1. **Enhanced Decision-making in Healthcare for Disease Prevention:** AI empowers healthcare providers to make informed decisions by analyzing vast amounts of patient data, including medical records, genetic information, lifestyle factors, and environmental data. AI algorithms

can uncover intricate patterns and correlations within complex datasets, enabling more accurate diagnoses, treatment plans, and disease prevention strategies.

2. **Predictive Modeling for Early Disease Detection:** AI-driven predictive analytics forecast disease risks and identify early warning signs by analyzing historical patient data. By recognizing subtle indicators and risk factors, AI algorithms enable healthcare professionals to intervene proactively, initiate preventive measures, and mitigate disease progression before symptoms manifest, thereby improving patient outcomes and reducing healthcare costs.

3. **Personalized Medicine and Treatment Strategies:** AI tailors personalized healthcare interventions based on individual patient profiles, genetic predispositions, and predictive analytics insights. By integrating patient-specific data with predictive models, healthcare providers can optimize treatment plans, predict treatment responses, and customize preventive strategies to address unique patient needs effectively.

4. **Optimization of Public Health Initiatives:** AI enhances public health efforts by analyzing population health data to forecast disease outbreaks, identify epidemiological trends, and allocate resources strategically. Predictive analytics enable health authorities to implement targeted interventions, vaccination campaigns, and healthcare policies that mitigate health risks, enhance community health outcomes, and promote public safety.

5. **Improved Operational Efficiency and Resource Allocation:** AI-driven predictive analytics optimize healthcare operational workflows by forecasting patient volumes, predicting resource demands, and improving healthcare resource allocation. By automating administrative tasks, streamlining patient scheduling, and optimizing hospital bed management, AI enhances operational efficiency, reduces wait times, and maximizes healthcare delivery capacity.

6. **Mitigation of Healthcare Risks and Regulatory Compliance:** AI aids in identifying potential healthcare risks, such as medication errors, patient safety concerns, and compliance violations, through advanced anomaly detection and real-time monitoring. AI-powered systems enhance regulatory compliance by alerting healthcare providers to deviations from protocols, ensuring adherence to healthcare standards, and safeguarding patient welfare and institutional reputation.

7. **Competitive Advantage and Innovation in Healthcare:** Healthcare organizations leveraging AI in predictive analytics gain a competitive edge by pioneering innovative healthcare solutions, advancing clinical research, and fostering collaborations in data-driven healthcare. By harnessing AI technologies, healthcare providers can lead industry advancements, attract top talent, and establish themselves as leaders in predictive medicine and disease prevention.

8. **Ethical Considerations and Patient Privacy:** The adoption of AI in predictive analytics necessitates ethical considerations, including patient consent, data privacy protections, and transparency in algorithmic decision-making. Upholding ethical standards ensures patient trust, maintains confidentiality of sensitive health information, and mitigates ethical implications associated with AI-driven healthcare innovations.

In summary, the integration of AI in predictive analytics and disease prevention represents a paradigm shift in healthcare delivery, offering unprecedented opportunities to enhance diagnostic accuracy, personalize patient care, and mitigate health risks proactively. By harnessing AI's predictive capabilities, healthcare providers can optimize healthcare outcomes, drive innovation, and forge a path towards a more efficient, equitable, and sustainable healthcare ecosystem.

Examples:

1. **Enhanced Decision-making in Healthcare:**

Company: Cerner

Example: Cerner uses AI-powered predictive analytics to assist healthcare providers in making informed decisions. Their platform analyzes patient data to predict disease progression, optimize treatment plans, and improve clinical outcomes through data-driven insights.

2. **Predictive Modeling for Early Disease Detection:**

Company: Tempus

Example: Tempus applies AI to genomic data analysis for early disease detection. Their platform uses machine learning algorithms to identify genetic markers associated with diseases like cancer, enabling proactive screening and personalized treatment strategies.

3. **Personalized Medicine and Treatment Strategies:**

Company: DeepMind Health

Example: DeepMind Health develops AI algorithms for personalized medicine by analyzing patient data and medical images. Their technology supports clinicians in tailoring treatment strategies based on individual patient profiles, improving treatment outcomes and patient care.

4. **Optimization of Public Health Initiatives:**

Company: BlueDot

Example: BlueDot utilizes AI-driven predictive analytics to monitor global health data and identify potential disease outbreaks. Their platform analyzes diverse datasets including travel patterns and climate data to optimize public health initiatives and mitigate the spread of infectious diseases.

5. **Improved Operational Efficiency and Resource Allocation:**

Company: KenSci

> **Example:** KenSci uses AI for healthcare predictive analytics to optimize operational efficiency. Their platform predicts patient outcomes, hospital readmissions, and resource needs, enabling healthcare providers to allocate resources effectively and reduce costs while maintaining quality of care.

6. **Mitigation of Healthcare Risks and Regulatory Compliance:**

> **Company: IBM Watson Health**
>
> **Example:** IBM Watson Health applies AI to healthcare risk management and regulatory compliance. Their solutions analyze clinical data to identify potential risks, ensure compliance with healthcare regulations, and improve patient safety through predictive analytics and decision support.

7. **Competitive Advantage and Innovation in Healthcare:**

> **Company: Anthem**
>
> **Example:** Anthem leverages AI in predictive analytics to gain a competitive advantage in healthcare. Their initiatives focus on using machine learning to predict healthcare trends, improve member health outcomes, and innovate in patient care delivery models.

8. **Ethical Considerations and Patient Privacy:**

> **Company: Verily (formerly Google Life Sciences)**
>
> **Example:** Verily addresses ethical considerations in AI-driven healthcare by prioritizing patient privacy and data security. Their AI algorithms for disease prevention and predictive analytics adhere to stringent ethical guidelines and regulatory standards to protect patient confidentiality and trust.

These examples demonstrate how various companies are leveraging AI in predictive analytics and disease prevention to enhance decision-making, detect diseases early, personalize medicine, optimize public health efforts, improve operational efficiency, ensure regulatory compliance, innovate in healthcare, and uphold ethical standards regarding patient privacy and data security.

3.1 Predictive Modeling for Disease Outbreaks

Artificial Intelligence (AI) is revolutionizing disease surveillance and outbreak prediction in healthcare, offering advanced capabilities that enhance preparedness, response, and management.

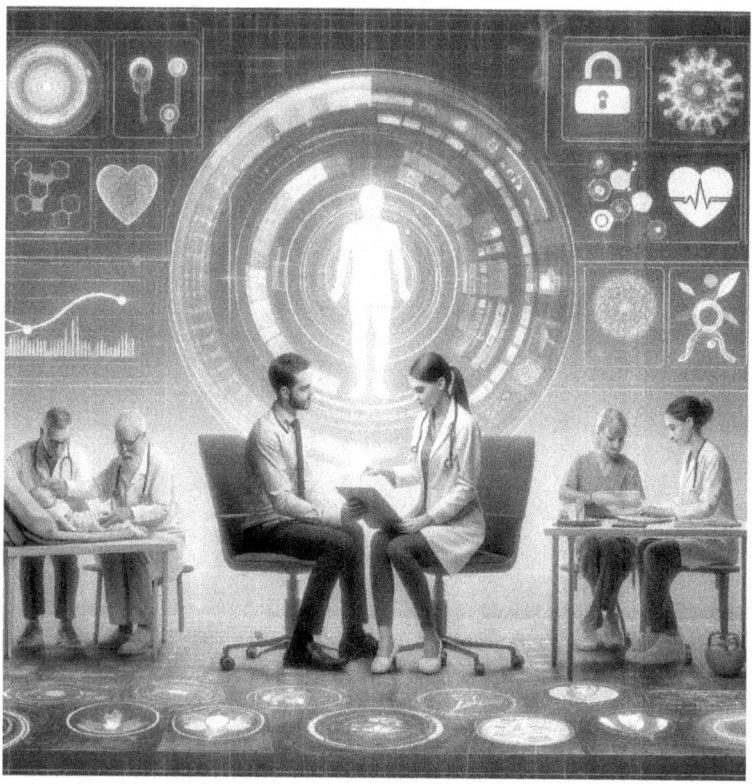

Here's why AI adoption is crucial in predicting and managing disease outbreaks:

1. **Enhanced Data-driven Decision-making:** AI enables healthcare organizations to analyze vast amounts of structured and unstructured data from various sources including patient records, demographic data, environmental factors, and global

health databases. AI algorithms can identify patterns, trends, and early indicators of disease outbreaks that may not be apparent through traditional methods. This data-driven approach enhances decision-making in public health responses and resource allocation.

2. **Early Detection and Rapid Response:** AI-powered predictive models can detect early signs of disease outbreaks by monitoring symptoms, geographic patterns, and population health data in real-time. This enables healthcare authorities to initiate timely interventions such as targeted vaccination campaigns, quarantine measures, and resource mobilization to mitigate the spread of infectious diseases.

3. **Optimization of Public Health Interventions:** AI enables healthcare systems to optimize public health interventions by predicting disease transmission dynamics and assessing the effectiveness of preventive measures. Machine learning algorithms can simulate scenarios to evaluate different intervention strategies, helping authorities to prioritize actions and allocate resources more effectively.

4. **Integration with Epidemiological Models:** AI enhances traditional epidemiological models by incorporating real-time data updates and adaptive learning capabilities. This integration improves the accuracy of disease forecasts, including epidemic curves, infection rates, and geographic spread predictions. Healthcare professionals can utilize these insights to implement proactive measures and mitigate the impact of outbreaks.

5. **Risk Assessment and Preparedness Planning:** AI facilitates proactive risk assessment by analyzing historical outbreak data, environmental factors, and population demographics. Predictive analytics help healthcare organizations to identify high-risk areas and vulnerable populations, allowing for targeted surveillance and preventive healthcare interventions.

6. **Enhanced Collaboration and Data Sharing:** AI-driven platforms facilitate collaboration among healthcare agencies, researchers, and international organizations by providing centralized data repositories and real-time analytics. This promotes knowledge sharing, early warning systems, and coordinated responses to global health threats.

7. **Cost-effective Resource Allocation:** AI algorithms optimize resource allocation by predicting disease burden and healthcare demand during outbreaks. This enables healthcare providers to allocate medical supplies, personnel, and facilities efficiently, minimizing shortages and optimizing response times.

8. **Continuous Learning and Adaptation:** AI systems continuously learn from new data inputs and feedback, improving predictive accuracy over time. Adaptive algorithms adjust models based on evolving disease patterns and emerging variants, ensuring resilience against future outbreaks and pandemics.

In summary, the adoption of AI in predictive modeling for disease outbreaks is essential for enhancing early detection, response planning, and resource management in healthcare. By leveraging AI technologies for data-driven decision-making, real-time surveillance, and collaborative efforts, healthcare organizations can effectively predict, monitor, and mitigate the impact of infectious diseases, safeguarding public health and ensuring timely interventions.

Examples:

1. **Enhanced Data-driven Decision-making:**

   Company: BlueDot

   Example: BlueDot utilizes predictive modeling and AI to enhance data-driven decision-making in disease outbreak scenarios. Their platform analyzes global health data, including travel patterns and epidemiological information, to predict and monitor infectious disease outbreaks such as COVID-19, enabling early intervention and response strategies.

2. **Early Detection and Rapid Response:**

   Company: Metabiota

   Example: Metabiota employs predictive modeling for early detection and rapid response to disease outbreaks. Their AI-driven platform integrates epidemiological data with environmental and socio-economic factors to forecast outbreaks, facilitating proactive public health interventions and mitigating health risks globally.

3. **Optimization of Public Health Interventions:**

   Company: HealthMap

   Example: HealthMap uses predictive modeling to optimize public health interventions during disease outbreaks. Their AI algorithms analyze diverse datasets, including news reports, social media, and official health reports, to provide real-time disease surveillance and inform targeted interventions for effective outbreak control.

4. **Integration with Epidemiological Models:**

   Company: Epistemix

   Example: Epistemix integrates predictive modeling with epidemiological models to simulate disease outbreaks.

Their platform uses AI to model disease transmission dynamics, assess intervention strategies, and forecast population-level health outcomes, supporting decision-makers in optimizing disease control measures.

5. **Risk Assessment and Preparedness Planning:**

Company: Epidemico (a subsidiary of Booz Allen Hamilton)

Example: Epidemico applies predictive modeling for risk assessment and preparedness planning in disease outbreaks. Their AI-powered tools analyze health data streams to assess population vulnerabilities, predict disease spread patterns, and support public health agencies in developing proactive preparedness strategies.

6. **Enhanced Collaboration and Data Sharing:**

Company: InSTEDD

Example: InSTEDD facilitates enhanced collaboration and data sharing through predictive modeling in disease outbreaks. Their AI-driven platforms enable real-time data integration from multiple sources, fostering cross-sectoral collaboration among healthcare providers, governments, and humanitarian organizations to improve outbreak response coordination.

7. **Cost-effective Resource Allocation:**

Company: Ubenwa

Example: Ubenwa uses predictive modeling for cost-effective resource allocation during disease outbreaks. Their AI algorithms analyze vocal biomarkers to predict neonatal asphyxia risk in newborns, enabling timely intervention and efficient allocation of healthcare resources in resource-constrained settings.

8. **Continuous Learning and Adaptation:**

Company: Verily (formerly Google Life Sciences)

> **Example**: Verily employs predictive modeling for continuous learning and adaptation in disease outbreaks. Their AI-driven platforms analyze real-time health data to detect emerging trends, refine predictive models, and adapt response strategies, supporting ongoing improvement in outbreak preparedness and response efforts.

These examples demonstrate how various companies and organizations leverage predictive modeling and AI in healthcare to enhance decision-making, detect disease outbreaks early, optimize public health interventions, integrate with epidemiological models, assess risks, facilitate collaboration, allocate resources efficiently, and continuously adapt to emerging health threats.

3.2 AI in Personalized Medicine and Risk Assessment

Artificial Intelligence (AI) is revolutionizing personalized medicine and risk assessment in healthcare, offering transformative benefits that improve patient outcomes, optimize treatment strategies, and enhance healthcare delivery.

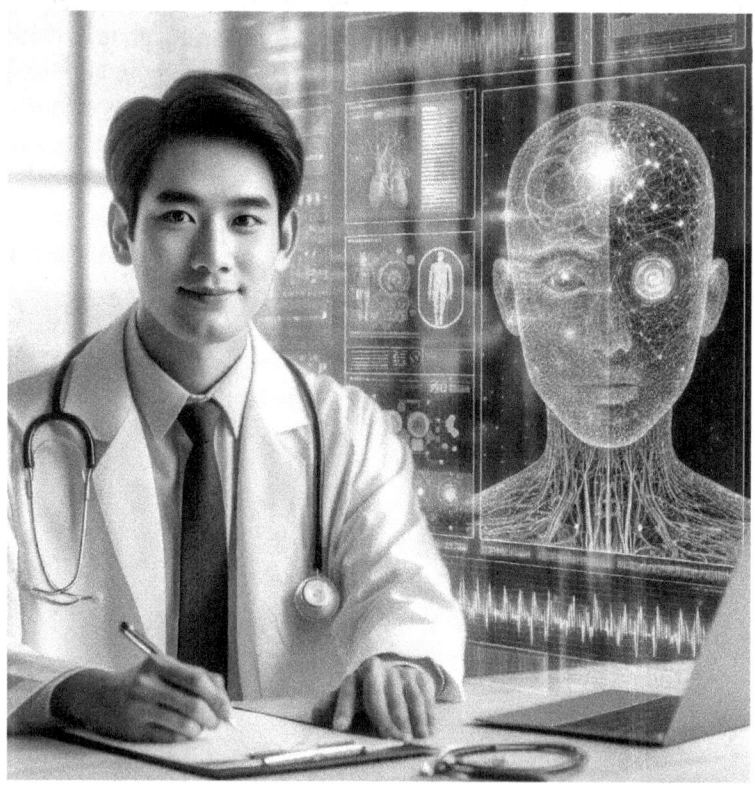

Here's why AI adoption is crucial in these domains:

1. **Enhanced Decision-making in Personalized Medicine:** AI enables healthcare providers to make data-driven decisions by analyzing comprehensive patient data including genomic information, medical history, lifestyle factors, and treatment outcomes. AI

algorithms identify complex patterns and correlations that guide personalized treatment plans tailored to individual patient profiles, optimizing therapeutic efficacy and patient satisfaction.

2. **Predictive Modeling for Disease Risk Assessment:** AI-powered predictive models analyze large datasets to assess disease risks based on genetic predispositions, environmental factors, and lifestyle behaviors. Machine learning algorithms predict disease onset, progression, and susceptibility, enabling proactive interventions and personalized preventive strategies to mitigate health risks before symptoms manifest.

3. **Precision Diagnosis and Treatment Planning:** AI enhances diagnostic accuracy by interpreting medical imaging scans, pathology reports, and molecular data with high precision. Deep learning algorithms detect subtle abnormalities and biomarkers, facilitating early disease detection and precise treatment planning customized to patient-specific characteristics and disease profiles.

4. **Optimization of Therapeutic Interventions:** AI-driven clinical decision support systems integrate patient data with medical knowledge and evidence-based guidelines to optimize treatment protocols. AI algorithms analyze real-time patient responses to therapies, predict treatment outcomes, and adjust interventions dynamically, ensuring personalized care delivery and therapeutic success.

5. **Personalized Drug Discovery and Development:** AI accelerates drug discovery processes by simulating molecular interactions, predicting drug efficacy, and identifying potential therapeutic targets. Machine learning algorithms analyze vast

biological datasets to discover novel drug candidates tailored to specific genetic mutations and disease mechanisms, advancing personalized medicine and innovative treatments.

6. **Improving Patient Outcomes and Quality of Life:** AI enhances patient outcomes by tailoring healthcare interventions to individual needs, preferences, and genetic predispositions. Personalized medicine approaches improve treatment effectiveness, reduce adverse effects, and enhance patient adherence to therapeutic regimens, ultimately improving quality of life and long-term health outcomes.

7. **Cost-effective Healthcare Delivery and Resource Allocation:** AI optimizes healthcare resource allocation by predicting patient care needs, hospitalization risks, and healthcare utilization patterns. Predictive analytics identify high-risk patient cohorts requiring intensive monitoring and intervention, enabling healthcare providers to allocate resources efficiently and manage healthcare costs effectively.

8. **Enhancing Regulatory Compliance and Patient Data Security:** AI-powered systems ensure compliance with healthcare regulations by safeguarding patient data privacy, maintaining data integrity, and detecting anomalies that may indicate security breaches or regulatory non-compliance. AI-driven cybersecurity measures protect patient information against unauthorized access and cyber threats, preserving trust and confidentiality in personalized healthcare settings.

In summary, the adoption of AI in personalized medicine and risk assessment is essential for advancing precision healthcare, improving treatment outcomes, and optimizing healthcare delivery. By leveraging AI technologies for personalized diagnostics, predictive modeling, and therapeutic optimization, healthcare providers can deliver tailored interventions, mitigate health risks, and enhance patient-centric care, ushering in a new era of personalized medicine.

Examples:

1. **Enhanced Decision-making in Personalized Medicine AI:**

   Company: Tempus Labs

   Example: Tempus Labs utilizes AI to enhance decision-making in personalized medicine. Their platform analyzes clinical and molecular data from patients to provide oncologists with insights for personalized treatment plans, improving treatment efficacy and patient outcomes.

2. **Predictive Modeling for Disease Risk Assessment with AI:**

   Company: Owkin

   Example: Owkin employs AI-driven predictive modeling for disease risk assessment. Their federated learning platform enables healthcare researchers to collaborate while preserving data privacy. AI algorithms analyze multi-modal data to predict disease progression and assess individualized risk profiles.

3. **Precision Diagnosis and Treatment Planning with AI:**

   Company: Paige

   Example: Paige uses AI for precision diagnosis and treatment planning in pathology. Their AI pathology software assists pathologists by analyzing digital pathology images to identify and classify cancerous tissues accurately, supporting personalized treatment strategies and improving patient outcomes.

4. **Optimization of Therapeutic Interventions with AI:**

> **Company: Mendel.ai**
>
> **Example:** Mendel.ai applies AI to optimize therapeutic interventions. Their platform uses natural language processing (NLP) and machine learning to extract and analyze clinical data from electronic health records (EHRs), aiding physicians in identifying suitable clinical trials and personalized treatment options for patients.

5. **Personalized Drug Discovery and Development with AI:**

> **Company: Insilico Medicine**
>
> **Example:** Insilico Medicine leverages AI for personalized drug discovery and development. Their AI-driven drug discovery platforms use generative adversarial networks (GANs) and reinforcement learning to design novel molecules and predict their biological activity, accelerating drug development timelines and improving drug efficacy.

6. **Improving Patient Outcomes and Quality of Life with AI:**

> **Company: Aktana**
>
> **Example:** Aktana enhances patient outcomes and quality of life with AI-driven personalized healthcare solutions. Their AI platform analyzes patient data, clinical guidelines, and treatment protocols to provide healthcare providers with personalized recommendations for patient care, improving treatment adherence and health outcomes.

7. **Cost-effective Healthcare Delivery and Resource Allocation with AI:**

> **Company: Komodo Health**
>
> **Example:** Komodo Health uses AI for cost-effective healthcare delivery and resource allocation. Their AI platform integrates real-world data from diverse sources to analyze patient populations, predict disease trends, and optimize healthcare resource allocation, enabling providers to deliver more efficient and targeted care.

8. **Enhancing Regulatory Compliance and Patient Data Security with AI:**

Company: Datavant
Example: Datavant enhances regulatory compliance and patient data security with AI-driven solutions. Their data integration and privacy platforms use advanced AI techniques to anonymize and securely link healthcare data across disparate sources while ensuring compliance with regulatory standards such as HIPAA, safeguarding patient privacy and data security.

These examples illustrate how various companies leverage AI technologies to advance personalized medicine, improve risk assessment, optimize therapeutic interventions, drive drug discovery, enhance patient outcomes, allocate healthcare resources efficiently, and ensure regulatory compliance in healthcare settings.

3.3 Early Detection and Prevention Strategies using AI

Artificial Intelligence (AI) is playing a pivotal role in revolutionizing early detection and prevention strategies in healthcare, offering transformative benefits that improve patient outcomes, reduce healthcare costs, and enhance public health.

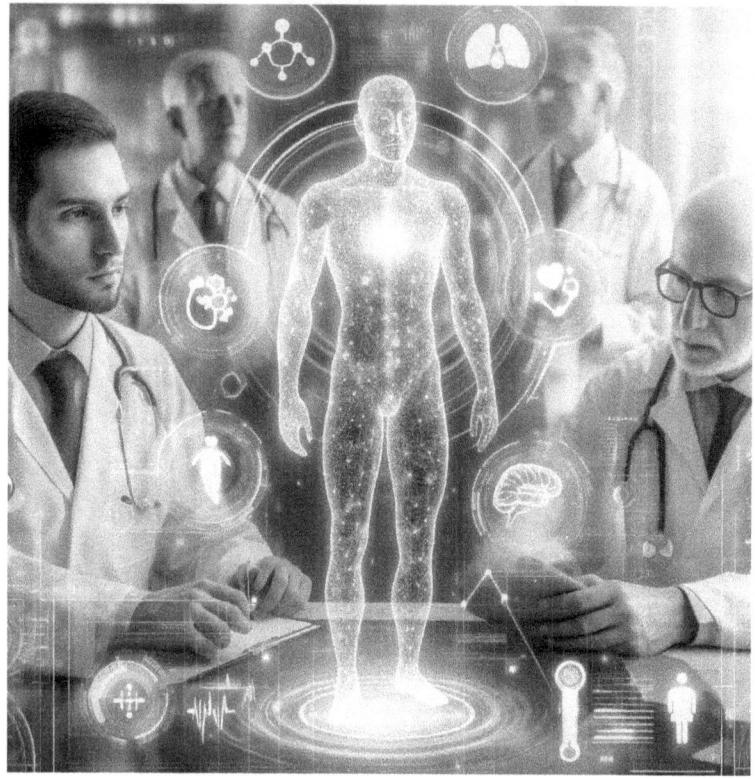

Here are key reasons why AI adoption is crucial in this domain:

1. **Enhanced Diagnostic Accuracy and Early Detection:** AI-powered diagnostic tools analyze complex medical data including imaging scans, genetic markers, and patient records with unparalleled accuracy. Machine learning algorithms detect subtle patterns and anomalies indicative of disease onset at early stages, enabling

healthcare providers to initiate timely interventions and improve treatment outcomes.

2. **Predictive Modeling for Disease Prevention:** AI algorithms leverage predictive analytics to assess individual and population health risks based on diverse data sources such as genetic predispositions, lifestyle factors, and environmental exposures. Predictive models identify high-risk cohorts susceptible to chronic diseases, allowing healthcare providers to implement personalized preventive measures and lifestyle interventions.

3. **Optimization of Screening Programs:** AI enhances screening programs by prioritizing at-risk populations for preventive screenings and early interventions. Machine learning algorithms analyze screening data to refine risk stratification models, improving screening efficiency and reducing unnecessary procedures while ensuring early detection of diseases such as cancer, cardiovascular conditions, and infectious diseases.

4. **Personalized Health Interventions:** AI-driven personalized medicine approaches tailor healthcare interventions to individual patient profiles and disease risks. AI algorithms integrate patient data with clinical guidelines and evidence-based practices to optimize treatment plans, enhance medication adherence, and mitigate health risks, ultimately improving patient outcomes and quality of life.

5. **Real-time Surveillance and Outbreak Prediction:** AI-powered surveillance systems monitor population health data in real-time, detecting disease outbreaks and epidemiological trends swiftly. Predictive analytics analyze demographic shifts, environmental factors, and social determinants of health to forecast disease spread, enabling proactive public health responses and resource allocation during emergencies.

6. **Cost-effective Healthcare Delivery and Resource Allocation:** AI optimizes healthcare resource allocation by predicting disease burdens, healthcare utilization

patterns, and patient care needs. Predictive analytics identify high-risk individuals requiring intensive management and preventive interventions, allowing healthcare providers to allocate resources efficiently, reduce hospital admissions, and manage healthcare costs effectively.

7. **Continuous Learning and Adaptation:** AI systems continuously learn from new data inputs and feedback, improving predictive accuracy and adapting to evolving healthcare challenges. Adaptive algorithms enhance decision support systems, enabling healthcare professionals to make informed decisions based on real-time insights and evidence-based practices.

8. **Regulatory Compliance and Data Security:** AI-driven healthcare platforms ensure compliance with regulatory standards by safeguarding patient data privacy, maintaining data integrity, and detecting potential security breaches. AI technologies implement robust cybersecurity measures to protect sensitive health information, ensuring regulatory compliance and maintaining patient trust in healthcare settings.

In summary, the adoption of AI in early detection and prevention strategies is essential for advancing healthcare outcomes, reducing disease burdens, and promoting population health. By leveraging AI technologies for enhanced diagnostic accuracy, predictive modeling, personalized interventions, and real-time surveillance, healthcare providers can achieve proactive disease management, improve patient care quality, and mitigate public health risks effectively.

Examples:

1. **Enhanced Diagnostic Accuracy and Early Detection with AI:**

   Company: Butterfly Network

   Example: Butterfly Network utilizes AI to enhance diagnostic accuracy and early detection. Their handheld ultrasound devices, powered by AI algorithms, assist healthcare providers in imaging interpretation and early diagnosis of various medical conditions, improving patient outcomes through timely interventions.

2. **Predictive Modeling for Disease Prevention with AI:**

    Company: ClosedLoop.ai

    Example: ClosedLoop.ai applies predictive modeling for disease prevention. Their healthcare AI platform analyzes patient data from EHRs and other sources to predict disease risks and recommend personalized preventive interventions, enabling healthcare providers to proactively manage patient health and reduce disease incidence.

3. **Optimization of Screening Programs with AI:**

    Company: Qure.ai

    Example: Qure.ai optimizes screening programs with AI-driven solutions. Their deep learning algorithms analyze medical imaging data (such as chest X-rays) to detect abnormalities indicative of diseases like tuberculosis and lung cancer, facilitating early detection and improving the efficiency of screening programs.

4. **Personalized Health Interventions with AI:**

    Company: Health Catalyst

    Example: Health Catalyst leverages AI for personalized health interventions. Their healthcare analytics platform integrates clinical and financial data to identify high-risk patient populations and recommend personalized interventions, improving patient engagement and health outcomes while reducing healthcare costs.

5. **Real-time Surveillance and Outbreak Prediction with AI:**

    Company: BlueDot

    Example: BlueDot uses AI for real-time surveillance and outbreak prediction. Their platform analyzes diverse data sources, including news reports and global travel patterns, to detect and predict infectious disease outbreaks worldwide, enabling early response and public health interventions to mitigate spread.

6. **Cost-effective Healthcare Delivery and Resource Allocation with AI:**

   Company: Apixio

   Example: Apixio facilitates cost-effective healthcare delivery and resource allocation with AI. Their AI platform extracts insights from unstructured healthcare data to optimize care management, improve care coordination, and allocate resources efficiently, enhancing operational efficiency and patient outcomes.

7. **Continuous Learning and Adaptation with AI:**

   Company: Gauss Surgical

   Example: Gauss Surgical enables continuous learning and adaptation with AI in healthcare. Their AI-powered blood monitoring technology monitors surgical blood loss in real-time, providing accurate measurements and actionable insights to clinicians for immediate decision-making and ongoing improvements in surgical outcomes.

8. **Regulatory Compliance and Data Security with AI:**

   Company: Ciitizen

   Example: Ciitizen ensures regulatory compliance and data security with AI-driven solutions. Their platform empowers patients to securely collect, manage, and share their medical records using AI to automate data organization and ensure compliance with privacy regulations such as HIPAA, safeguarding patient data integrity and security.

These examples demonstrate how AI technologies are applied across various aspects of early detection and prevention strategies in healthcare, from enhancing diagnostic accuracy and predictive modeling to optimizing healthcare delivery and ensuring regulatory compliance.

4. AI in Treatment and Patient Care

Artificial Intelligence (AI) is revolutionizing the healthcare industry by enhancing treatment methodologies and optimizing patient care through innovative applications.

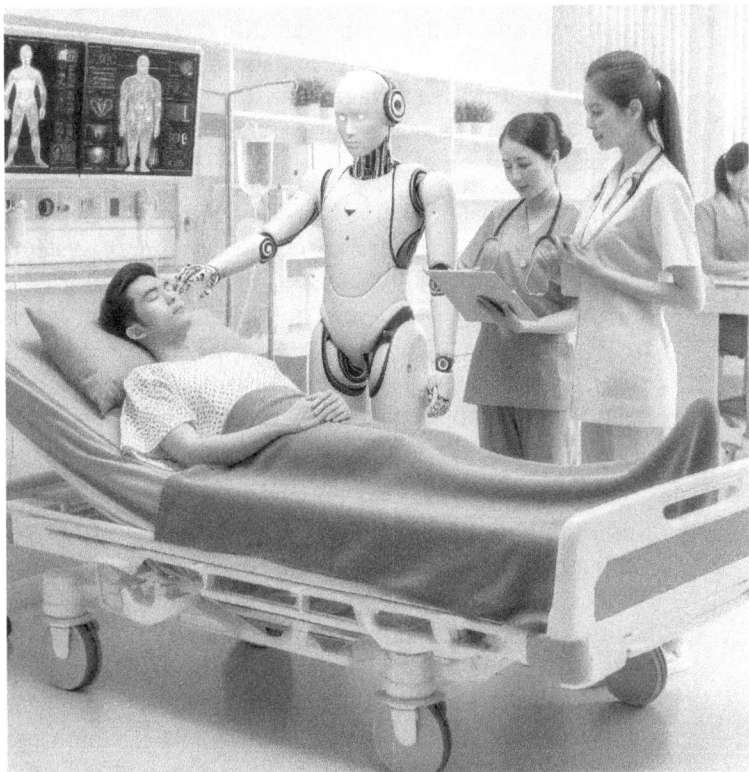

Here's an exploration of why AI adoption in treatment and patient care is crucial:

1. **Enhanced Treatment Decision-making:** AI empowers healthcare providers to make data-driven treatment decisions by analyzing extensive patient data, including medical records, diagnostic images, genetic profiles, and real-time physiological data. AI algorithms can uncover patterns and correlations within complex datasets that aid in diagnosing diseases, predicting treatment outcomes,

and personalizing therapies based on individual patient profiles.

2. **Personalized Medicine and Treatment Plans:** AI enables personalized medicine by tailoring treatment plans to individual patient characteristics, genetic predispositions, and responsiveness to therapies. Machine learning algorithms analyze patient data to predict optimal treatments, dosage adjustments, and potential adverse reactions, thereby improving treatment efficacy and patient outcomes.

3. **Support for Clinical Decision Support Systems (CDSS):** AI-driven clinical decision support systems enhance healthcare provider decision-making by integrating evidence-based guidelines, patient data analytics, and medical literature. CDSS powered by AI assist in diagnosing complex cases, recommending treatment protocols, and alerting healthcare professionals to potential risks or drug interactions, thereby improving clinical accuracy and patient safety.

4. **Remote Patient Monitoring and Telehealth:** AI facilitates remote patient monitoring through wearable devices and IoT-enabled sensors that capture real-time health data, such as vital signs, glucose levels, and activity patterns. AI algorithms analyze continuous monitoring data to detect health fluctuations, trigger alerts for intervention, and enable proactive healthcare management, enhancing patient autonomy and reducing hospital readmissions.

5. **Improving Operational Efficiency and Workflow Optimization:** AI optimizes healthcare operational workflows by automating administrative tasks, streamlining patient scheduling, and enhancing resource allocation. AI-powered predictive analytics forecast patient flow, bed occupancy rates, and staffing needs, thereby reducing wait times, optimizing hospital resources, and improving overall operational efficiency.

6. **Enhancing Patient Engagement and Satisfaction:** AI technologies improve patient engagement by providing personalized health insights, educational resources, and interactive communication channels. Virtual health assistants powered by natural language processing (NLP) and chatbots offer patient support, answer queries, and deliver appointment reminders, enhancing patient satisfaction, adherence to treatment plans, and continuity of care.

7. **Facilitating Medical Imaging and Diagnosis:** AI algorithms enhance diagnostic accuracy in medical imaging by analyzing radiological images, pathology slides, and scans to detect abnormalities, quantify disease progression, and assist in early detection of conditions such as cancer or neurological disorders. AI-powered imaging tools improve diagnostic confidence, reduce interpretation errors, and expedite treatment initiation, ultimately improving patient outcomes.

8. **Ethical Considerations and Patient Privacy:** The adoption of AI in treatment and patient care necessitates adherence to ethical guidelines, including patient consent, data privacy protections, and transparency in AI decision-making processes. Upholding ethical standards ensures patient trust, safeguards sensitive health information, and mitigates ethical implications associated with AI-driven healthcare innovations.

In summary, AI adoption in treatment and patient care represents a transformative shift towards personalized, efficient, and patient-centric healthcare delivery. By leveraging AI technologies, healthcare providers can optimize treatment decisions, enhance clinical workflows, improve patient outcomes, and ultimately redefine standards of care in the modern healthcare landscape.

Example:

1. **Enhanced Treatment Decision-making:**

Company/Software: Memorial Sloan Kettering Cancer Center (MSKCC), IBM Watson for Oncology

Example: MSKCC utilizes IBM Watson for Oncology to assist oncologists in treatment decision-making by providing AI-driven treatment recommendations based on patient-specific data and clinical guidelines. This enhances the accuracy and consistency of treatment plans across their network.

2. **Personalized Medicine and Treatment Plans:**

Company/Software: Deep Genomics

Example: Deep Genomics uses AI to analyze genetic data and patient health records to develop personalized treatment plans for genetic disorders. Their platform integrates genomic information with clinical data to recommend targeted therapies tailored to individual patients.

3. **Support for Clinical Decision Support Systems (CDSS):**

Company/Software: Cerner Corporation, Healhixx

Example: Cerner's Healhixx CDSS incorporates AI algorithms to provide real-time clinical decision support. It analyzes patient data, medical literature, and best practices to assist healthcare providers in making informed treatment decisions and optimizing patient outcomes.

4. **Remote Patient Monitoring and Telehealth:**

Company/Software: Biofourmis, Current Health

Example: Biofourmis and Current Health utilize AI-powered remote monitoring systems that collect continuous physiological data from patients. AI algorithms analyze this data to detect early signs of deterioration, enabling timely intervention and adjustment of treatment plans in telehealth settings.

5. **Improving Operational Efficiency and Workflow Optimization:**

Company/Software: Olive, Google DeepMind Health

Example: Olive's AI platform automates administrative tasks and streamlines healthcare workflows. It optimizes scheduling, resource allocation, and inventory management, improving operational efficiency in hospitals and clinics. Google DeepMind Health develops AI solutions that enhance healthcare delivery by analyzing patient data to improve treatment planning and resource utilization.

6. **Enhancing Patient Engagement and Satisfaction:**

Company/Software: Myia Health, Ada Health

Example: Myia Health and Ada Health employ AI to provide personalized health insights and recommendations directly to patients. Their platforms engage patients in self-management, adherence to treatment plans, and lifestyle modifications, thereby enhancing patient satisfaction and health outcomes.

7. **Facilitating Medical Imaging and Diagnosis:**

Company/Software: Zebra Medical Vision, Aidoc

Example: Zebra Medical Vision and Aidoc develop AI-powered medical imaging analysis tools. These tools assist radiologists in interpreting imaging scans (e.g., CT, MRI) by detecting abnormalities and providing diagnostic insights, which support accurate treatment planning and patient management.

8. **Ethical Considerations and Patient Privacy:**

Company/Example: Johns Hopkins Hospital, MedWhat

Example: Johns Hopkins Hospital integrates AI-driven treatment planning systems while prioritizing patient privacy and ethical considerations. They ensure compliance with regulations such as HIPAA and implement transparent AI algorithms that maintain patient confidentiality and consent. MedWhat addresses ethical concerns by developing AI systems that prioritize patient safety and

> privacy, ensuring that treatment recommendations are based on ethical principles and patient-centric care.

These examples illustrate how various companies and technologies are leveraging AI to enhance different aspects of treatment planning and recommendations in healthcare while addressing ethical considerations and patient privacy concerns.

4.1 AI-driven Treatment Planning and Recommendations

Artificial Intelligence (AI) is revolutionizing healthcare by enhancing treatment planning and recommendations through innovative applications.

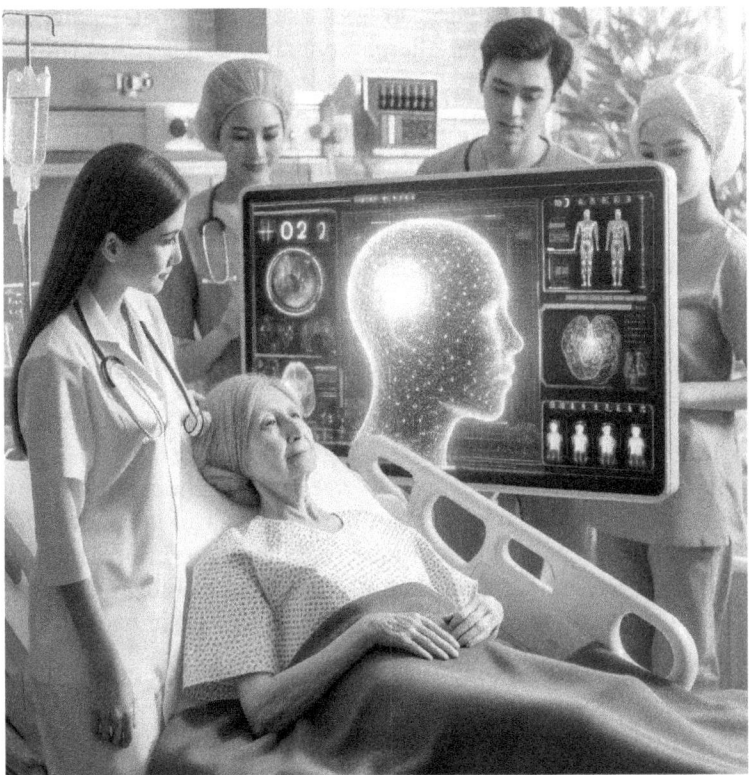

Here's an exploration of why AI adoption in treatment planning and recommendations is crucial:

1. **Enhanced Treatment Decision-making:** AI facilitates data-driven treatment decisions by analyzing comprehensive patient data, including medical records, genetic information, diagnostic images, and real-time physiological data. AI algorithms uncover patterns and correlations within large datasets that assist healthcare providers in diagnosing diseases, predicting treatment

outcomes, and personalizing therapies based on individual patient profiles.

2. **Personalized Treatment Plans:** AI enables personalized medicine by tailoring treatment plans to the unique characteristics of each patient. Machine learning algorithms analyze patient data to predict optimal treatments, adjust dosages, and anticipate potential adverse reactions, thereby enhancing treatment efficacy and patient safety.

3. **Clinical Decision Support Systems (CDSS):** AI-powered CDSS integrate patient data with evidence-based guidelines and medical literature to support healthcare professionals in diagnosing complex conditions, recommending treatment protocols, and identifying risks or contraindications. These systems improve clinical accuracy, reduce diagnostic errors, and streamline decision-making processes.

4. **Optimization of Therapeutic Strategies:** AI algorithms optimize therapeutic strategies by analyzing treatment response data from diverse patient populations. By identifying treatment patterns that lead to successful outcomes, AI enables continuous refinement of therapeutic approaches, fostering innovation in disease management and improving patient care pathways.

5. **Predictive Analytics for Treatment Outcomes:** AI leverages predictive analytics to forecast treatment outcomes based on historical data and patient characteristics. By identifying predictive markers and treatment response patterns, AI assists healthcare providers in making proactive decisions, adjusting treatment plans, and optimizing patient recovery trajectories.

6. **Integration with Medical Imaging and Diagnostics:** AI enhances diagnostic accuracy by analyzing medical imaging scans, pathology slides, and other diagnostic data. AI algorithms detect subtle anomalies, quantify disease progression, and provide quantitative insights that

aid in early detection and treatment planning, thereby improving clinical outcomes and patient prognosis.

7. **Patient-Centric Care and Engagement:** AI technologies support patient-centric care by providing personalized health insights, treatment recommendations, and educational resources. Virtual health assistants powered by AI enhance patient engagement through interactive communication, remote monitoring capabilities, and timely intervention alerts, promoting adherence to treatment plans and improving patient satisfaction.

8. **Ethical Considerations and Regulatory Compliance:** The adoption of AI in treatment planning requires adherence to ethical standards, patient consent protocols, and regulatory compliance frameworks. Ensuring transparency in AI algorithms, protecting patient privacy, and addressing ethical implications are essential to maintaining trust, safeguarding sensitive health information, and upholding ethical standards in AI-driven healthcare innovations.

In summary, AI adoption in treatment planning and recommendations empowers healthcare providers to deliver personalized, efficient, and evidence-based care. By leveraging AI technologies, healthcare organizations can optimize treatment decisions, enhance clinical workflows, improve patient outcomes, and redefine standards of care in the evolving landscape of modern healthcare delivery.

Example:
1. **Enhanced Treatment Decision-making:**

> **Company/Software: Memorial Sloan Kettering Cancer Center (MSKCC), IBM Watson for Oncology**
>
> **Example:** MSKCC uses IBM Watson for Oncology to assist clinicians in making treatment decisions. Watson analyzes patient data (e.g., medical records, research papers) to provide evidence-based treatment

recommendations, improving the accuracy and speed of decision-making in cancer care.

2. **Personalized Treatment Plans:**

   Company/Software: Tempus Labs, DeepMind Health

   Example: Tempus Labs leverages AI to analyze genomic and clinical data to create personalized treatment plans for cancer patients. Their platform integrates molecular data with patient health records to tailor therapies based on individual genetic profiles and disease characteristics.

3. **Clinical Decision Support Systems (CDSS):**

   Company/Software: Cerner Corporation, Epic Systems

   Example: Cerner and Epic integrate AI into their clinical decision support systems (CDSS) to assist healthcare providers in diagnosing and treating patients. These systems analyze patient data in real-time to recommend appropriate treatments and interventions based on medical guidelines and best practices.

4. **Optimization of Therapeutic Strategies:**

   Company/Software: AiCure, AiCure

   Example: AiCure uses AI-powered medication adherence platforms to optimize therapeutic strategies for patients. The system monitors medication intake through facial recognition and behavioral analytics, providing insights that help healthcare providers adjust treatment plans to improve patient outcomes.

5. **Predictive Analytics for Treatment Outcomes:**

   Company/Software: Gauss Surgical, PhysIQ

   Example: Gauss Surgical applies AI to predict surgical outcomes by analyzing real-time blood loss data during operations. Their platform, Triton, uses machine learning to enhance decision-making in surgery, helping clinicians anticipate and mitigate potential complications for better patient outcomes.

6. **Integration with Medical Imaging and Diagnostics:**

> **Company/Software: Aidoc, Zebra Medical Vision**
>
> **Example:** Aidoc and Zebra Medical Vision develop AI algorithms that analyze medical imaging scans (e.g., CT, MRI) to aid radiologists in detecting abnormalities and making accurate diagnoses. These tools integrate with existing imaging systems to improve diagnostic accuracy and guide treatment planning.

7. **Patient-Centric Care and Engagement:**

> **Company/Software: Conversa Health, Lark Health**
>
> **Example:** Conversa Health and Lark Health utilize AI-driven virtual health assistants to engage patients in self-management and treatment adherence. These platforms provide personalized guidance, monitor patient progress, and facilitate communication between patients and healthcare providers to enhance patient-centric care.

8. **Ethical Considerations and Regulatory Compliance:**

> **Company/Example: Verily (formerly Google Life Sciences), MedWhat**
>
> **Example:** Verily incorporates ethical considerations into their AI-driven healthcare solutions by prioritizing patient privacy and data security. Their platforms adhere to regulations such as HIPAA and GDPR to ensure that patient data is handled responsibly and transparently. MedWhat addresses ethical concerns by developing AI systems that prioritize patient safety and privacy, ensuring that treatment recommendations are based on ethical principles and patient consent.

These examples demonstrate how AI is being integrated into various aspects of healthcare to improve treatment planning and recommendations while addressing ethical considerations and regulatory compliance.

4.2 Virtual Health Assistants and Chatbots

Artificial Intelligence (AI) has significantly transformed the healthcare industry, particularly through the adoption of Virtual Health Assistants (VHAs) and chatbots.

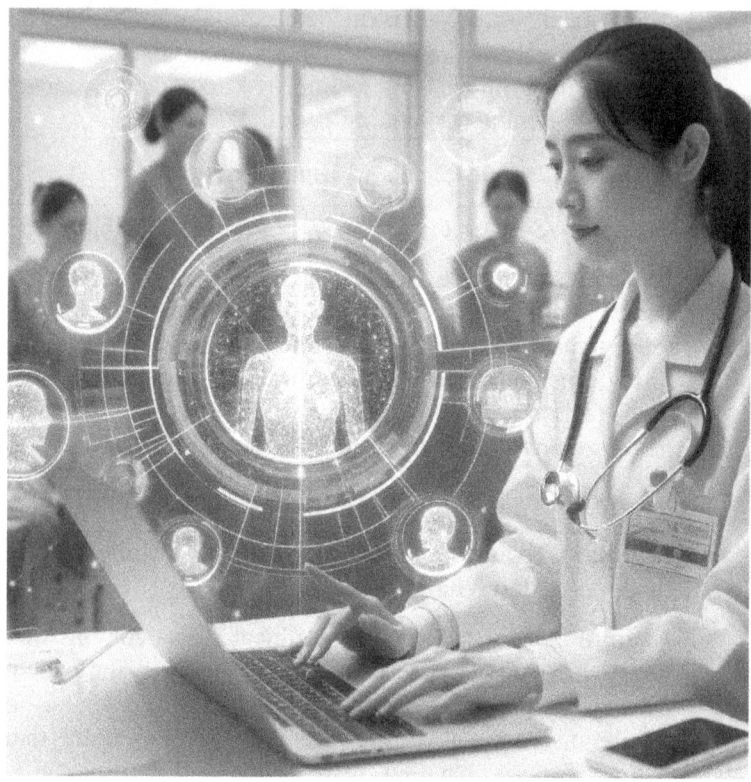

Here's an exploration of why AI adoption in VHAs and chatbots is crucial:

1. **Enhanced Patient Interaction and Engagement:** VHAs and chatbots powered by AI enhance patient interaction by providing personalized assistance, answering queries, and offering medical advice based on individual health data. These AI-driven solutions improve patient engagement by offering 24/7 accessibility, responding promptly to inquiries, and delivering consistent

information, thereby enhancing overall patient satisfaction.

2. **Efficient Appointment Scheduling and Management:** AI-powered chatbots streamline appointment scheduling processes by autonomously managing appointments, sending reminders, and rescheduling bookings based on patient preferences and healthcare provider availability. This automation reduces administrative burden, optimizes clinic workflows, minimizes no-show rates, and improves operational efficiency.

3. **Personalized Health Monitoring and Management:** VHAs equipped with AI monitor patients' health metrics in real-time, analyze data trends, and provide personalized health management recommendations. AI algorithms detect anomalies, alert healthcare providers to potential issues, and offer timely interventions, thereby supporting proactive disease management and improving patient outcomes.

4. **Health Education and Empowerment:** AI-driven VHAs and chatbots deliver educational content, preventive healthcare tips, and lifestyle recommendations tailored to individual patient profiles. By promoting health literacy, encouraging adherence to treatment plans, and fostering self-care practices, these AI solutions empower patients to take proactive steps toward maintaining their health and well-being.

5. **Integration with Telemedicine and Remote Monitoring:** AI facilitates seamless integration of VHAs and chatbots with telemedicine platforms, enabling virtual consultations, remote monitoring of chronic conditions, and remote diagnostic assessments. This integration expands access to healthcare services, improves care continuity, and enhances patient convenience, particularly in underserved or remote regions.

6. **Data-driven Insights for Healthcare Providers:** AI analyzes patient interactions, health records, and

treatment outcomes to generate actionable insights for healthcare providers. By identifying care gaps, predicting patient health risks, and recommending evidence-based interventions, AI-driven VHAs support clinical decision-making, improve care coordination, and enhance healthcare delivery efficiency.

7. **Compliance with Healthcare Regulations and Ethical Standards:** AI adoption in VHAs and chatbots necessitates adherence to healthcare regulations, patient confidentiality laws, and ethical guidelines. Ensuring data security, maintaining transparency in AI algorithms, obtaining informed consent, and addressing ethical considerations are essential to building patient trust and fostering responsible AI deployment in healthcare settings.

8. **Continuous Improvement and Adaptability:** AI-powered VHAs continuously learn from patient interactions, feedback, and data updates to enhance performance, refine response accuracy, and adapt to evolving healthcare needs. By leveraging machine learning capabilities, VHAs improve over time, incorporate new medical knowledge, and evolve as indispensable tools in modern healthcare delivery.

In summary, AI adoption in Virtual Health Assistants and chatbots revolutionizes patient care by enhancing interaction, improving operational efficiency, supporting clinical decision-making, and empowering patients to actively manage their health. By harnessing AI technologies, healthcare organizations can deliver patient-centered care, optimize resource utilization, and redefine healthcare delivery standards in an increasingly digital and interconnected healthcare ecosystem.

Examples:

1. **Enhanced Patient Interaction and Engagement:**

   Company/Software: Babylon Health, Your.MD

   Example: Babylon Health's AI-powered chatbot interacts with patients to provide personalized health advice based on symptoms and medical history. It engages users in proactive health management and connects them with healthcare professionals when necessary, enhancing patient engagement.

2. **Efficient Appointment Scheduling and Management:**

Company/Software: Qventus, Medumo (acquired by Philips)

Example: Qventus uses AI to optimize hospital operations, including appointment scheduling. Their platform analyzes real-time data to predict patient flow and manage resources efficiently, reducing wait times and improving patient satisfaction. Medumo's platform, now part of Philips, sends automated reminders and instructions to patients, improving appointment adherence and operational efficiency.

3. **Personalized Health Monitoring and Management:**

Company/Software: Conversa Health, Lark Health

Example: Conversa Health develops virtual health assistants that monitor patients' health status and provide personalized guidance. Their platform engages patients in chronic disease management through automated check-ins and symptom tracking, fostering proactive healthcare management.

4. **Health Education and Empowerment:**

Company/Software: Ada Health, Buoy Health

Example: Ada Health's AI-driven platform educates users about symptoms, conditions, and treatment options. It empowers patients to make informed healthcare decisions by providing personalized health assessments and educational content based on individual health data.

5. **Integration with Telemedicine and Remote Monitoring:**

Company/Software: TytoCare, Amwell

Example: TytoCare integrates AI-powered virtual health assistants with telemedicine solutions for remote consultations. Their platform enables patients to conduct self-examinations and share data with healthcare providers via video consultations, enhancing remote monitoring capabilities.

6. **Data-driven Insights for Healthcare Providers:**

Company/Software: Infermedica, HealthTap

Example: Infermedica's AI-driven chatbot analyzes symptoms and medical history to generate preliminary diagnoses and treatment recommendations. It provides healthcare providers with data-driven insights that support clinical decision-making and improve diagnostic accuracy.

7. **Compliance with Healthcare Regulations and Ethical Standards:**

Company/Software: Nuance Communications (Dragon Medical), Welltok

Example: Nuance Communications' Dragon Medical AI ensures compliance with healthcare regulations by securely transcribing patient-doctor interactions. It maintains patient confidentiality and data privacy while supporting accurate documentation and regulatory compliance. Welltok's virtual health assistant adheres to ethical standards by providing evidence-based health recommendations and promoting wellness programs that prioritize patient privacy and consent.

8. **Continuous Improvement and Adaptability:**

Company/Software: Gyant, Buoy Health

Example: Gyant's virtual health assistant continuously learns from interactions to improve responses and adapt to user needs. It uses AI to refine its diagnostic capabilities and enhance the user experience, ensuring that patients receive accurate information and support over time.

These examples illustrate how various companies are leveraging virtual health assistants and chatbots in healthcare to improve patient interaction, streamline operations, enhance monitoring and management, and ensure compliance with ethical and regulatory standards.

4.3 AI in Remote Monitoring and Telehealth

Artificial Intelligence (AI) is revolutionizing the healthcare industry, particularly in remote monitoring and telehealth, offering transformative benefits to patients and healthcare providers alike.

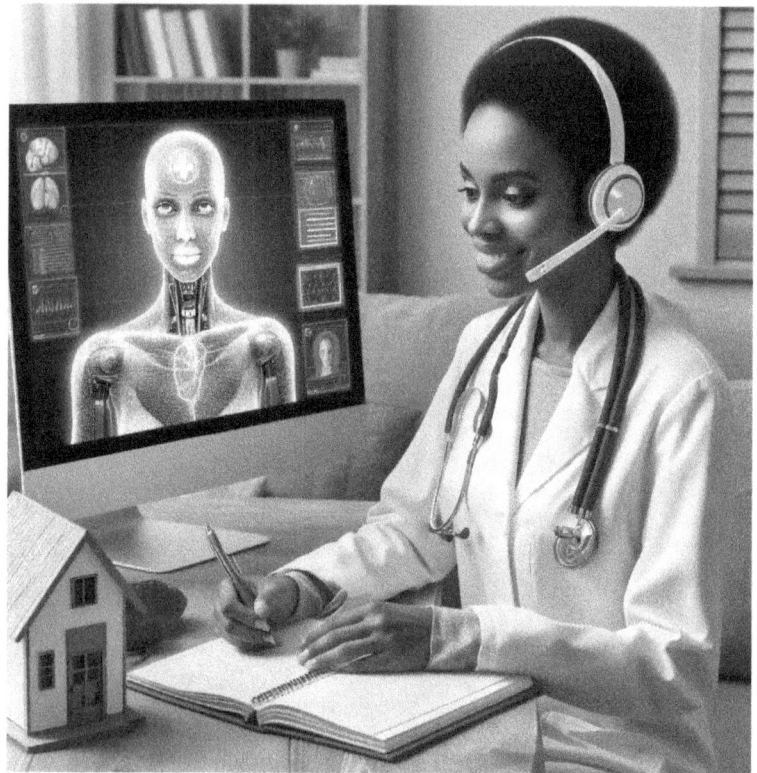

Here's an exploration of why AI adoption in remote monitoring and telehealth is crucial:

1. **Enhanced Patient Monitoring and Management:** AI-powered remote monitoring systems enable continuous tracking of patients' vital signs, health metrics, and adherence to treatment plans from remote locations. These systems analyze real-time data, detect abnormalities, and alert healthcare providers to intervene

promptly, thereby improving patient outcomes and reducing the need for frequent hospital visits.

2. **Optimized Healthcare Delivery and Accessibility:** AI facilitates virtual consultations and remote diagnostic assessments through telehealth platforms. This accessibility eliminates geographical barriers, expands healthcare access to underserved populations, and enhances care continuity for patients with chronic conditions or limited mobility. AI-driven telehealth improves healthcare delivery efficiency by minimizing waiting times and optimizing healthcare resource allocation.

3. **Personalized Treatment Plans and Predictive Insights:** AI algorithms analyze patient data, medical histories, and diagnostic images to generate personalized treatment recommendations. By leveraging machine learning, AI predicts disease progression, identifies risk factors, and recommends preventive measures tailored to individual patient profiles. These predictive insights empower healthcare providers to deliver proactive and targeted care interventions, thereby enhancing treatment outcomes and patient satisfaction.

4. **Efficient Resource Management and Cost Savings:** AI-driven telehealth solutions optimize healthcare resource utilization by reducing unnecessary hospital visits, mitigating emergency room overcrowding, and lowering healthcare operational costs. Telehealth consultations powered by AI enhance clinic workflows, increase appointment scheduling efficiency, and minimize administrative burdens, resulting in significant cost savings for healthcare organizations.

5. **Data Security and Regulatory Compliance:** AI in remote monitoring and telehealth ensures robust data security measures and compliance with healthcare regulations (e.g., HIPAA in the United States). AI algorithms encrypt patient data, monitor access controls, and adhere to privacy standards to safeguard sensitive

health information. Maintaining data integrity and patient confidentiality builds trust among patients and healthcare providers, supporting widespread adoption of AI-driven telehealth solutions.

6. **Continuous Monitoring and Early Intervention:** AI-enabled remote monitoring systems track patient health metrics continuously, providing real-time insights into physiological changes and treatment responses. AI algorithms detect health deterioration early, predict adverse events, and notify healthcare providers to initiate timely interventions. This proactive approach minimizes disease progression, reduces hospital readmissions, and improves overall patient care quality.

7. **Enhanced Patient Engagement and Satisfaction:** AI-powered telehealth platforms enhance patient engagement through personalized health education, interactive symptom tracking tools, and virtual health coaching. These tools empower patients to actively participate in their healthcare management, adhere to treatment plans, and make informed lifestyle choices. Improved patient engagement fosters stronger patient-provider relationships and enhances overall healthcare satisfaction.

8. **Integration with Wearable Devices and IoT:** AI integrates with wearable devices and Internet of Things (IoT) sensors to collect real-time patient data, such as heart rate, blood pressure, and activity levels. These interconnected technologies enable seamless data transmission to AI platforms, facilitating comprehensive health monitoring and enabling healthcare providers to make data-driven decisions based on objective physiological metrics.

In summary, AI adoption in remote monitoring and telehealth transforms healthcare delivery by enhancing patient monitoring, optimizing resource utilization, and facilitating personalized treatment approaches. By leveraging AI technologies, healthcare organizations can overcome geographical barriers, improve clinical outcomes, and redefine the future of healthcare delivery in an increasingly digital and interconnected world.

Examples:

1. **Enhanced Patient Monitoring and Management:**

   Company/Software: Current Health, Biofourmis

   Example: Current Health utilizes AI to monitor patients remotely through wearable devices. Their platform analyzes physiological data in real-time to detect early signs of deterioration and alerts healthcare providers for timely intervention, improving patient monitoring and management.

2. **Optimized Healthcare Delivery and Accessibility:**

   Company/Software: TytoCare, Amwell

   Example: TytoCare integrates AI into remote monitoring solutions that enable patients to conduct virtual exams with healthcare providers. Their platform enhances healthcare accessibility by facilitating remote consultations and reducing the need for in-person visits, optimizing healthcare delivery.

3. **Personalized Treatment Plans and Predictive Insights:**

   Company/Software: Lark Health, Ada Health

   Example: Lark Health's AI-driven platform offers personalized coaching and health monitoring. It analyzes patient data to provide tailored treatment plans and predictive insights, empowering patients to manage chronic conditions remotely with personalized guidance.

4. **Efficient Resource Management and Cost Savings:**

   Company/Software: VivaLNK, Current Health

   Example: VivaLNK's wearable sensors and AI-powered analytics optimize resource management in remote patient monitoring. By remotely monitoring vital signs and health metrics, healthcare providers can allocate resources more efficiently, reducing costs associated with unnecessary hospital visits and readmissions.

5. **Data Security and Regulatory Compliance:**

   Company/Software: Philips Healthcare, BioIntelliSense

   Example: Philips Healthcare ensures data security and regulatory compliance in remote monitoring with AI-powered solutions. Their platforms, such as BioIntelliSense, adhere to healthcare regulations like HIPAA, protecting patient data while enabling continuous health monitoring and remote care management.

6. **Continuous Monitoring and Early Intervention:**

   Company/Software: Biofourmis, Current Health

   Example: Biofourmis employs AI to continuously monitor patients remotely and detect deviations from baseline health indicators. Their platform supports early intervention by alerting healthcare providers to potential health risks, improving patient outcomes through proactive care.

7. **Enhanced Patient Engagement and Satisfaction:**

   Company/Software: Conversa Health, Wellth

   Example: Conversa Health's virtual health assistant engages patients in remote monitoring programs through personalized interactions. It delivers educational content, tracks health progress, and encourages adherence to treatment plans, enhancing patient engagement and satisfaction.

8. **Integration with Wearable Devices and IoT:**

   Company/Software: BioIntelliSense, Qualcomm Life

   Example: BioIntelliSense integrates AI with wearable devices and IoT solutions for remote monitoring. Their platform collects real-time health data from wearables, applies AI analytics for health insights, and transmits data

> securely to healthcare providers, facilitating comprehensive remote patient monitoring and telehealth services.

These examples highlight how AI is integrated into remote monitoring and telehealth solutions to enhance patient care, improve healthcare delivery efficiency, ensure data security, and promote patient engagement while complying with regulatory standards.

5. AI in Drug Discovery and Development

Artificial Intelligence (AI) is revolutionizing the pharmaceutical and biotech industries by accelerating drug discovery and development processes.

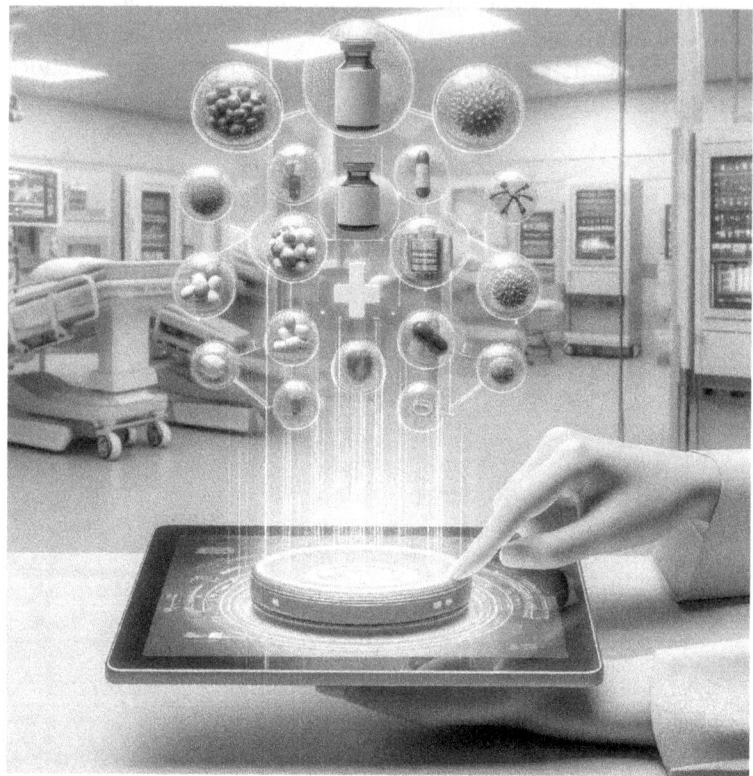

Here's an exploration of why AI adoption in drug discovery and development is crucial:

1. **Enhanced Decision-making in Drug Design:** AI enables pharmaceutical researchers to analyze vast datasets of molecular structures, biological targets, and clinical trial results. AI algorithms identify complex patterns and correlations that guide rational drug design, leading to the creation of novel compounds with optimized therapeutic properties. This data-driven approach enhances decision-making at early stages of drug development.

2. **Process Automation and Efficiency:** AI-powered automation streamlines various stages of drug discovery, including virtual screening, lead optimization, and toxicity prediction. By automating repetitive tasks such as compound screening and molecular docking, AI reduces manual effort and accelerates the identification of potential drug candidates. This efficiency gains significant time savings in the drug development timeline.

3. **Personalized Medicine and Targeted Therapies:** AI facilitates the identification of biomarkers and patient subpopulations most likely to benefit from specific treatments. Machine learning algorithms analyze genetic data, patient profiles, and clinical outcomes to predict individual responses to therapies. This personalized medicine approach tailors treatments to patients' genetic and physiological characteristics, improving treatment efficacy and patient outcomes.

4. **Predictive Analytics and Insights:** AI-driven predictive analytics analyze extensive biological and clinical data to forecast drug efficacy, safety profiles, and adverse effects. By integrating diverse data sources and utilizing deep learning models, AI predicts drug-drug interactions, pharmacokinetics, and potential side effects early in the development process. These insights inform strategic decisions and mitigate risks associated with clinical trials.

5. **Accelerated Clinical Trials and Regulatory Approval:** AI optimizes clinical trial design by identifying eligible patient cohorts, predicting trial outcomes, and optimizing trial protocols. Natural language processing (NLP) algorithms extract insights from scientific literature and regulatory documents, aiding in protocol development and submission. AI expedites regulatory approval processes by providing robust data-driven evidence of drug safety and efficacy.

6. **Competitive Advantage and Innovation:** Organizations leveraging AI in drug discovery gain a competitive edge by reducing development costs, shortening timelines, and

increasing the success rate of drug candidates. AI-driven innovations enable biotech firms to explore new therapeutic areas, repurpose existing drugs, and develop breakthrough treatments that address unmet medical needs, positioning them as leaders in the pharmaceutical market.

7. **Scalability and Cost Savings:** AI technologies scale drug discovery operations by handling large volumes of genomic, proteomic, and clinical data. Cloud-based AI platforms facilitate collaboration among global research teams and academic institutions, enabling seamless data sharing and analysis. Scalable AI solutions reduce operational costs associated with laboratory experiments and computational modeling, optimizing resource allocation.

8. **Risk Mitigation and Compliance:** AI enhances drug safety and regulatory compliance by predicting potential adverse reactions and ensuring adherence to global pharmacovigilance standards. AI algorithms monitor real-world patient data to detect post-marketing drug safety signals and assess long-term treatment outcomes. This proactive risk mitigation strategy safeguards patient health and reinforces regulatory compliance throughout the drug lifecycle.

In summary, AI adoption in drug discovery and development transforms traditional approaches by enhancing decision-making, accelerating innovation, and optimizing resource utilization. By leveraging AI technologies, pharmaceutical companies can expedite the delivery of safe and effective therapies, improve patient outcomes, and address global healthcare challenges with unprecedented efficiency and precision.

Examples:
1. **Enhanced Decision-making in Drug Design:**

   Company/Software: Atomwise, Insilico Medicine

   Example: Atomwise uses AI to predict the binding of small molecules to proteins, accelerating drug discovery. Their platform analyzes molecular structures to identify potential drug candidates and optimize their effectiveness against specific diseases, enhancing decision-making in drug design.

2. **Process Automation and Efficiency:**

   Company/Software: XtalPi, BenchSci

   Example: XtalPi applies AI to predict drug properties and optimize drug formulation processes. Their platform automates molecular simulations and experimental design, improving efficiency in drug discovery and development by reducing the need for physical experiments and accelerating time to market.

3. **Personalized Medicine and Targeted Therapies:**

   Company/Software: Tempus Labs, Deep Genomics

   Example: Tempus Labs integrates AI with genomic data to develop personalized cancer therapies. Their platform analyzes genetic profiles to identify biomarkers and predict treatment responses, enabling targeted therapies that improve patient outcomes in oncology and other disease areas.

4. **Predictive Analytics and Insights:**

   Company/Software: BenevolentAI, Recursion Pharmaceuticals

   Example: BenevolentAI uses AI to analyze biomedical data and generate predictive insights for drug discovery. Their platform identifies novel drug targets and repurposes existing compounds by mining vast datasets, accelerating the discovery of treatments for complex diseases.

5. **Accelerated Clinical Trials and Regulatory Approval:**

   Company/Software: Saama Technologies, Mendel.ai

   Example: Saama Technologies leverages AI to optimize clinical trial processes and data analysis. Their platform accelerates patient recruitment, monitors trial progress in real-time, and predicts outcomes, streamlining regulatory approval and reducing time to market for new drugs.

6. **Competitive Advantage and Innovation:**

   Company/Software: Insilico Medicine, Numerate

   Example: Insilico Medicine pioneers AI-driven drug discovery by leveraging generative models and reinforcement learning. Their platform designs novel molecules with specific properties, providing pharmaceutical companies with a competitive edge in innovation and accelerating breakthroughs in drug development.

7. **Scalability and Cost Savings:**

   Company/Software: Recursion Pharmaceuticals, Cyclica

   Example: Recursion Pharmaceuticals uses AI for high-throughput screening of drug candidates across biological models. Their platform scales experimental capacity and reduces costs by automating image analysis and data interpretation, enhancing scalability in drug discovery programs.

8. **Risk Mitigation and Compliance:**

   Company/Software: Certara, Collaborative Drug Discovery (CDD Vault)

   Example: Certara employs AI to assess drug safety and predict potential adverse effects during preclinical and clinical development stages. Their platform integrates computational modeling with regulatory compliance, mitigating risks and ensuring adherence to safety standards throughout the drug discovery process.

These examples demonstrate how AI is transforming drug discovery and development by enhancing decision-making, automating processes, enabling personalized medicine, and improving efficiency while addressing regulatory compliance and ensuring patient safety.

5.1 Accelerating Drug Discovery with AI

Artificial Intelligence (AI) is reshaping the landscape of drug discovery and development, offering significant advantages to pharmaceutical and biotech industries.

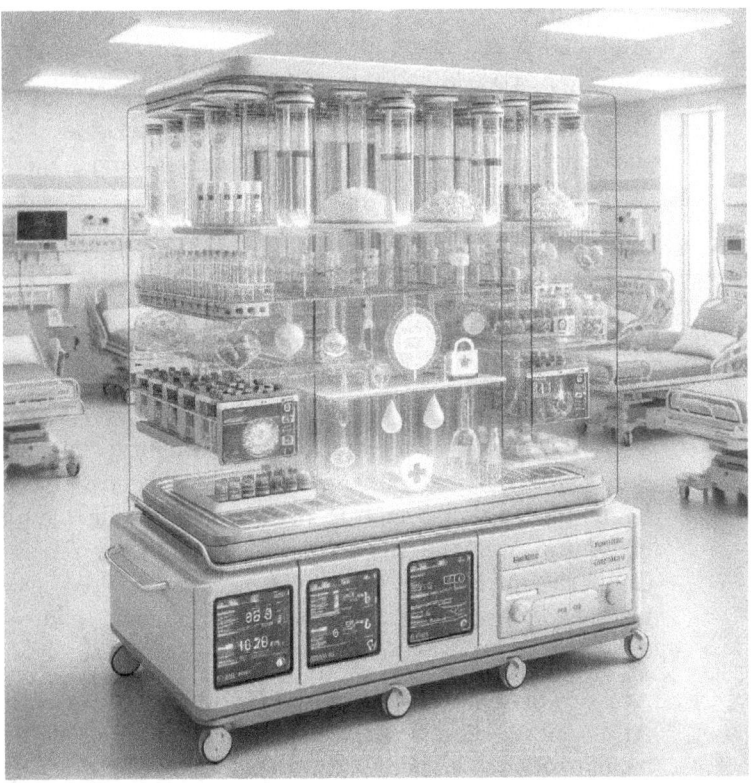

Here's an exploration of why AI adoption in accelerating drug discovery is crucial:

1. **Enhanced Decision-making in Compound Screening:** AI algorithms enable high-throughput screening of vast chemical libraries to identify potential drug candidates efficiently. By analyzing molecular structures, AI predicts binding affinities and pharmacological properties, guiding researchers to prioritize compounds with higher therapeutic potential. This data-driven approach enhances decision-making in early-stage drug discovery.

2. **Process Automation and Efficiency:** AI-powered automation streamlines various stages of drug discovery, from virtual screening to lead optimization. Machine learning models expedite compound selection by predicting bioactivity and toxicity profiles, reducing the time and resources required for experimental validation. Automation improves efficiency, accelerates timelines, and lowers costs associated with preclinical research.

3. **Personalized Medicine and Targeted Therapies:** AI facilitates the identification of biomarkers and patient subpopulations most likely to respond to specific treatments. By integrating genomic and clinical data, AI predicts treatment outcomes and tailors therapies to individual genetic profiles. This personalized medicine approach enhances treatment efficacy, minimizes adverse effects, and supports precision healthcare initiatives.

4. **Predictive Analytics and Insights:** AI-driven predictive analytics leverage integrated biological data to forecast drug efficacy, safety, and pharmacokinetics. Deep learning algorithms analyze diverse datasets, including genomics, proteomics, and clinical records, to predict drug-drug interactions and adverse reactions. Predictive insights inform decision-making throughout clinical development, enhancing trial design and patient safety.

5. **Accelerated Clinical Trials and Regulatory Approval:** AI optimizes clinical trial design by identifying eligible patient cohorts, predicting trial outcomes, and optimizing protocol parameters. Natural language processing (NLP) algorithms extract insights from scientific literature and real-world evidence, supporting regulatory submissions and accelerating approval processes. AI-driven evidence generation enhances regulatory compliance and expedites market entry.

6. **Competitive Advantage and Innovation:** Organizations adopting AI in drug discovery gain a competitive edge by accelerating the identification and optimization of drug candidates. AI-driven innovations enable

biopharmaceutical firms to explore novel therapeutic targets, repurpose existing drugs, and develop breakthrough treatments for unmet medical needs. AI fosters innovation, enhances pipeline diversification, and strengthens market positioning.

7. **Scalability and Cost Savings:** Cloud-based AI platforms facilitate collaborative research and data sharing among global teams, enhancing scalability and resource efficiency. AI technologies handle large-scale data integration and analysis, supporting scalable drug discovery operations without significant infrastructure investments. Cost-effective AI solutions reduce experimental costs and optimize resource allocation across research facilities.

8. **Risk Mitigation and Compliance:** AI enhances drug safety and regulatory compliance by predicting potential adverse events and ensuring adherence to pharmacovigilance standards. AI algorithms monitor real-world patient data to detect safety signals, assess treatment outcomes, and support post-marketing surveillance. Proactive risk management strategies mitigate regulatory risks and safeguard patient health throughout the drug lifecycle.

In summary, AI adoption in drug discovery accelerates innovation, enhances decision-making, and optimizes resource utilization in pharmaceutical research. By leveraging AI technologies, biotech companies can expedite the development of safe and effective therapies, improve patient outcomes, and address global health challenges with unprecedented efficiency and precision.

Examples:
1. **Enhanced Decision-making in Compound Screening:**

Company/Software: Atomwise, Insilico Medicine
Example: Atomwise uses AI to screen millions of compounds against specific disease targets. Their platform predicts molecular interactions and identifies promising

drug candidates, enhancing decision-making in compound screening and accelerating drug discovery.

2. **Process Automation and Efficiency:**

Company/Software: XtalPi, BenchSci

Example: XtalPi integrates AI into drug discovery workflows to automate molecular simulations and optimize experimental design. Their platform accelerates process efficiency by predicting drug properties and formulation processes, reducing the time and resources required for drug development.

3. **Personalized Medicine and Targeted Therapies:**

Company/Software: Tempus Labs, Deep Genomics

Example: Tempus Labs applies AI to analyze genomic data and develop personalized cancer therapies. Their platform identifies biomarkers and predicts treatment responses, enabling targeted therapies that improve patient outcomes and accelerate the adoption of precision medicine.

4. **Predictive Analytics and Insights:**

Company/Software: BenevolentAI, Recursion Pharmaceuticals

Example: BenevolentAI uses AI to analyze biomedical data and generate predictive insights for drug discovery. Their platform identifies novel drug targets and repurposes existing compounds by mining large datasets, accelerating the discovery of treatments for complex diseases.

5. **Accelerated Clinical Trials and Regulatory Approval:**

Company/Software: Saama Technologies, Mendel.ai

Example: Saama Technologies leverages AI to optimize clinical trial processes and data analysis. Their platform accelerates patient recruitment, monitors trial progress in real-time, and predicts outcomes, streamlining regulatory approval and reducing time to market for new drugs.

6. **Competitive Advantage and Innovation:**

> **Company/Software: Insilico Medicine, Numerate**
>
> **Example:** Insilico Medicine pioneers AI-driven drug discovery by leveraging generative models and reinforcement learning. Their platform designs novel molecules with specific properties, providing pharmaceutical companies with a competitive edge in innovation and accelerating breakthroughs in drug development.

7. **Scalability and Cost Savings:**

> **Company/Software: Recursion Pharmaceuticals, Cyclica**
>
> **Example:** Recursion Pharmaceuticals applies AI for high-throughput screening of drug candidates across biological models. Their platform scales experimental capacity and reduces costs by automating image analysis and data interpretation, enhancing scalability in drug discovery programs.

8. **Risk Mitigation and Compliance:**

> **Company/Software: Certara, Collaborative Drug Discovery (CDD Vault)**
>
> **Example:** Certara employs AI to assess drug safety and predict potential adverse effects during preclinical and clinical development. Their platform integrates computational modeling with regulatory compliance, mitigating risks and ensuring adherence to safety standards throughout the drug discovery process.

These examples illustrate how AI is revolutionizing drug discovery and development by improving decision-making, automating processes, enabling personalized medicine, and accelerating clinical trials while addressing regulatory compliance and ensuring patient safety.

5.2 AI in Clinical Trials and Research

Artificial Intelligence (AI) is revolutionizing the landscape of clinical trials and research, offering substantial benefits to the pharmaceutical, biotechnology, and healthcare sectors.

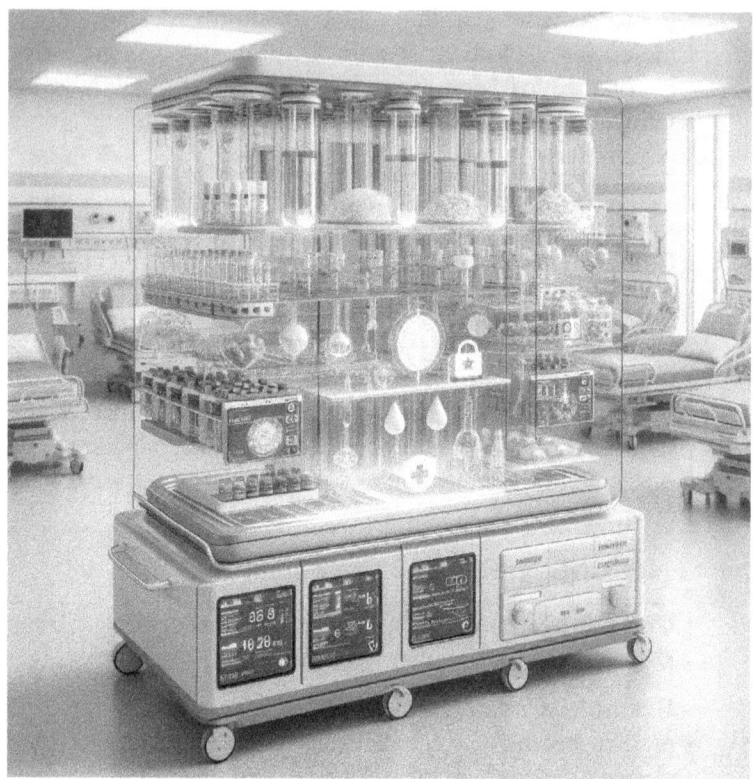

Here's an exploration of why AI adoption in clinical trials and research is crucial:

1. **Enhanced Decision-making in Trial Design:** AI empowers researchers to make data-driven decisions by analyzing vast datasets from previous trials, patient records, and biomedical literature. AI algorithms identify patterns in patient demographics, disease progression, and treatment outcomes, enabling optimized trial designs that enhance statistical power and reduce sample size requirements.

2. **Process Automation and Efficiency:** AI-driven automation accelerates various aspects of clinical trials, from patient recruitment to data analysis. Natural language processing (NLP) tools extract insights from electronic health records (EHRs) and medical literature, automating data collection and streamlining regulatory compliance. Automated workflows reduce administrative burden, enhance operational efficiency, and expedite trial timelines.

3. **Improved Patient Stratification and Personalized Medicine:** AI analyzes molecular, genomic, and clinical data to stratify patients based on biomarkers and disease subtypes. Machine learning models predict patient responses to treatments, facilitating personalized therapy selection and adaptive trial designs. By tailoring interventions to individual patient profiles, AI enhances treatment efficacy, reduces adverse events, and supports precision medicine initiatives.

4. **Enhanced Productivity and Innovation:** AI tools augment researchers' capabilities by automating routine tasks, such as image analysis and data integration across multiple platforms. This frees researchers to focus on complex analyses, hypothesis testing, and innovative trial methodologies. AI-driven innovation fosters novel approaches to drug discovery, biomarker identification, and therapeutic development, driving scientific breakthroughs.

5. **Predictive Analytics and Insights:** AI enables predictive modeling to forecast trial outcomes, patient adherence, and protocol deviations. Deep learning algorithms analyze real-time data streams from wearable devices and patient-reported outcomes, predicting clinical endpoints and treatment responses. Predictive analytics inform adaptive trial protocols, optimize resource allocation, and mitigate risks associated with trial conduct.

6. **Competitive Advantage and Market Leadership:** Organizations leveraging AI in clinical trials gain a

competitive edge by accelerating trial timelines and reducing costs associated with drug development. AI-driven insights expedite regulatory submissions, enhance market access strategies, and support lifecycle management of therapeutic products. By embracing AI-driven innovation, companies maintain leadership in therapeutic areas and market segments.

7. **Scalability and Cost Savings:** Cloud-based AI platforms facilitate scalable data processing and secure collaboration among global research teams. AI technologies handle large-scale data integration, ensuring data integrity and regulatory compliance across multicenter trials. Scalable AI solutions optimize resource utilization, reduce trial costs, and facilitate rapid expansion into emerging markets and therapeutic indications.

8. **Risk Mitigation and Compliance:** AI enhances trial safety and regulatory compliance by detecting adverse events, protocol deviations, and data anomalies in real time. AI-powered algorithms monitor patient safety data, identify early warning signs of adverse reactions, and support pharmacovigilance efforts. Proactive risk management strategies mitigate regulatory risks, safeguard patient welfare, and uphold ethical standards in clinical research.

In summary, AI adoption in clinical trials and research accelerates innovation, enhances decision-making, and optimizes resource utilization in drug development. By leveraging AI technologies, pharmaceutical and biotech companies can expedite the delivery of safe and effective therapies, improve patient outcomes, and address unmet medical needs with unprecedented efficiency and precision.

Examples:

1. **Enhanced Decision-making in Trial Design:**

Company/Software: Owkin, Deep 6 AI

> **Example:** Owkin uses AI to analyze patient data and biomarkers to optimize clinical trial design. Their platform integrates real-world evidence with clinical data to enhance decision-making, improving trial efficiency and accelerating drug development timelines.

2. **Process Automation and Efficiency:**

   > **Company/Software: Clinerion, Medidata (Acorn AI)**
   >
   > **Example:** Medidata's Acorn AI leverages AI to automate clinical trial processes such as patient recruitment and data analysis. Their platform uses predictive analytics to streamline trial operations, reduce manual tasks, and enhance overall efficiency in clinical research.

3. **Improved Patient Stratification and Personalized Medicine:**

   > **Company/Software: Tempus Labs, Deep 6 AI**
   >
   > **Example:** Tempus Labs applies AI to genomic data to stratify patients based on molecular profiles for clinical trials. Their platform identifies biomarkers and predicts treatment responses, enabling personalized medicine approaches that improve patient outcomes and trial success rates.

4. **Enhanced Productivity and Innovation:**

   > **Company/Software: AiCure, AiCRO**
   >
   > **Example:** AiCure uses AI-powered computer vision to monitor patient adherence and behavior during clinical trials. Their platform enhances productivity by automating data collection and analysis, fostering innovation in trial methodologies and improving trial outcomes.

5. **Predictive Analytics and Insights:**

   > **Company/Software: Saama Technologies, Mendel.ai**
   >
   > **Example:** Saama Technologies employs AI to analyze clinical trial data and predict patient outcomes. Their platform uses machine learning to generate insights,

optimize trial protocols, and predict recruitment challenges, improving decision-making and accelerating trial timelines.

6. **Competitive Advantage and Market Leadership:**

   Company/Software: Deep 6 AI, Clinerion

   Example: Deep 6 AI enables healthcare organizations to leverage AI for patient recruitment in clinical trials. Their platform uses natural language processing to identify eligible patients from electronic health records, providing a competitive advantage in trial recruitment and enhancing market leadership.

7. **Scalability and Cost Savings:**

   Company/Software: Medidata (Acorn AI), Clinerion

   Example: Medidata's Acorn AI improves scalability in clinical trials by automating data management and analysis. Their platform reduces trial costs and timelines by leveraging AI to optimize resource allocation, streamline operations, and enhance trial scalability.

8. **Risk Mitigation and Compliance:**

   Company/Software: IBM Watson Health, Veeva Systems

   Example: IBM Watson Health uses AI to ensure compliance and mitigate risks in clinical trials. Their platform enhances data integrity, monitors regulatory requirements, and automates audit processes, ensuring adherence to ethical standards and regulatory compliance throughout the research process.

These examples demonstrate how AI technologies are transforming clinical trials and research by improving decision-making, automating processes, enabling personalized medicine, and enhancing overall efficiency while addressing regulatory compliance and patient safety concerns.

5.3 Personalized Drug Development and Precision Medicine

Artificial Intelligence (AI) is reshaping the landscape of drug development and precision medicine, offering transformative opportunities for pharmaceutical companies, biotech firms, and healthcare providers.

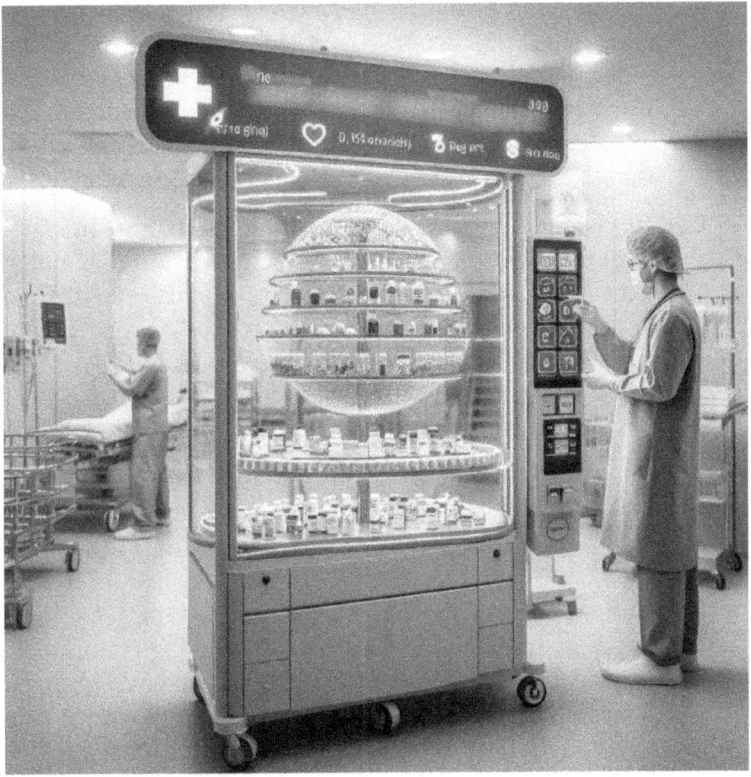

Here's a detailed exploration of why AI adoption in personalized drug development and precision medicine is crucial:

1. **Enhanced Decision-making in Drug Discovery:** AI empowers pharmaceutical researchers to make data-driven decisions by analyzing vast datasets encompassing genomics, proteomics, and clinical data. AI algorithms can uncover intricate patterns in disease mechanisms, biomarker identification, and therapeutic targets that

human analysis may overlook. This capability accelerates the drug discovery process, enhances target validation, and improves the success rate of clinical trials.

2. **Process Automation and Efficiency:** AI-driven automation streamlines various stages of drug development, from target identification to lead optimization and preclinical testing. Machine learning algorithms analyze molecular structures, predict compound interactions, and simulate drug efficacy, reducing the time and cost associated with experimental research. Automated workflows in data integration and experimental design optimize resource allocation, mitigate risks, and expedite regulatory submissions.

3. **Improved Patient Stratification and Personalized Treatment:** AI algorithms analyze patient data, including genetic profiles, biomarkers, and clinical records, to stratify populations into subgroups based on disease susceptibility and treatment response. This enables the delivery of targeted therapies tailored to individual patient profiles, optimizing treatment outcomes while minimizing adverse effects. AI-powered predictive models predict patient responses to therapies, supporting adaptive treatment strategies and enhancing patient-centric care delivery.

4. **Enhanced Productivity and Innovation:** AI tools augment researchers' capabilities by automating labor-intensive tasks such as data mining, image analysis, and pattern recognition in biomedical research. By freeing up researchers from routine tasks, AI fosters innovation in therapeutic modalities, drug delivery systems, and diagnostic technologies. AI-driven innovation accelerates the development of breakthrough therapies and promotes collaboration across multidisciplinary research teams.

5. **Predictive Analytics and Insights:** AI enables predictive modeling to forecast patient outcomes, disease progression, and treatment efficacy based on real-time data streams from wearable devices and remote

monitoring platforms. Predictive analytics support early intervention strategies, optimize clinical trial designs, and facilitate evidence-based decision-making in treatment selection and patient management. AI-driven insights from longitudinal patient data enhance post-market surveillance and support lifecycle management of therapeutic products.

6. **Competitive Advantage and Market Leadership:** Organizations leveraging AI in personalized drug development gain a competitive edge by accelerating the translation of scientific discoveries into clinical applications. AI-driven insights into patient subpopulations and treatment responses inform market access strategies, support regulatory approvals, and differentiate products in competitive markets. By harnessing AI-driven innovation, companies maintain leadership in therapeutic areas and drive market penetration in precision medicine.

7. **Scalability and Cost Savings:** Cloud-based AI platforms facilitate scalable data processing, secure data sharing, and collaborative research efforts across global networks of healthcare providers and research institutions. AI technologies optimize resource utilization, reduce operational costs, and enable rapid scalability in clinical trial recruitment and data management. Scalable AI solutions support cost-effective deployment of personalized therapies and expand access to precision medicine in diverse patient populations.

8. **Risk Mitigation and Compliance:** AI enhances regulatory compliance by automating documentation, monitoring adverse events, and detecting protocol deviations in clinical trials. AI-powered algorithms ensure data integrity, patient confidentiality, and adherence to regulatory guidelines, enhancing trial safety and ethical standards. Proactive risk management strategies mitigate compliance risks, safeguard patient welfare, and uphold trust in personalized medicine initiatives.

In summary, AI adoption in personalized drug development and precision medicine accelerates innovation, enhances patient outcomes, and addresses unmet medical needs with unprecedented efficiency and precision. By leveraging AI technologies, pharmaceutical and healthcare organizations can transform therapeutic discovery, optimize treatment strategies, and deliver personalized care that improves health outcomes and quality of life for patients worldwide.

Examples:

1. **Enhanced Decision-making in Drug Discovery:**

   Company/Software: Insilico Medicine, BenevolentAI

   Example: Insilico Medicine uses AI to accelerate drug discovery through deep learning models that predict molecular properties and interactions. Their platform enhances decision-making by identifying potential drug candidates and optimizing personalized treatment options based on genomic and clinical data.

2. **Process Automation and Efficiency:**

   Company/Software: Berg Health, Atomwise

   Example: Atomwise applies AI to automate virtual screening of drug compounds against disease targets. Their platform uses machine learning to analyze molecular structures and predict binding affinity, streamlining drug discovery processes and improving efficiency in personalized medicine development.

3. **Improved Patient Stratification and Personalized Treatment:**

   Company/Software: Tempus Labs, SOPHiA GENETICS

   Example: Tempus Labs integrates AI to analyze clinical and genomic data for patient stratification in clinical trials. Their platform uses machine learning to identify biomarkers and predict treatment responses, enabling personalized therapies and improving patient outcomes in precision medicine.

4. **Enhanced Productivity and Innovation:**

Company/Software: XtalPi, Numerate

Example: XtalPi leverages AI-driven quantum mechanics to simulate drug molecular structures and properties. Their platform accelerates innovation by predicting drug formulation and optimizing manufacturing processes, enhancing productivity in personalized drug development.

5. **Predictive Analytics and Insights:**

Company/Software: Owkin, Mendel.ai

Example: Owkin uses AI to analyze patient data and predict treatment outcomes in clinical trials. Their platform applies federated learning to protect patient privacy while generating predictive insights, guiding personalized treatment decisions and improving clinical trial efficiency.

6. **Competitive Advantage and Market Leadership:**

Company/Software: BenevolentAI, Recursion Pharmaceuticals

Example: BenevolentAI applies AI to uncover novel drug targets and pathways. Their platform enhances competitive advantage by accelerating drug discovery and development, positioning companies at the forefront of personalized medicine innovation and market leadership.

7. **Scalability and Cost Savings:**

Company/Software: BenchSci, GNS Healthcare

Example: GNS Healthcare uses AI to analyze real-world evidence and clinical data for predictive modeling in drug development. Their platform improves scalability by optimizing trial designs and reducing costs associated with patient recruitment and treatment optimization in personalized medicine.

8. **Risk Mitigation and Compliance:**

Company/Software: IBM Watson Health, Saama Technologies

Example: IBM Watson Health employs AI to ensure regulatory compliance and mitigate risks in personalized medicine research. Their platform enhances data integrity, monitors regulatory requirements, and automates audit processes, ensuring adherence to ethical standards and regulatory compliance throughout drug development.

These examples illustrate how AI technologies are revolutionizing personalized drug development and precision medicine by enhancing decision-making, automating processes, improving patient outcomes, and addressing regulatory and ethical considerations in drug discovery and development.

6. AI in Healthcare Operations and Management

Artificial Intelligence (AI) is revolutionizing healthcare operations and management, offering transformative benefits for hospitals, clinics, pharmaceutical companies, and healthcare providers.

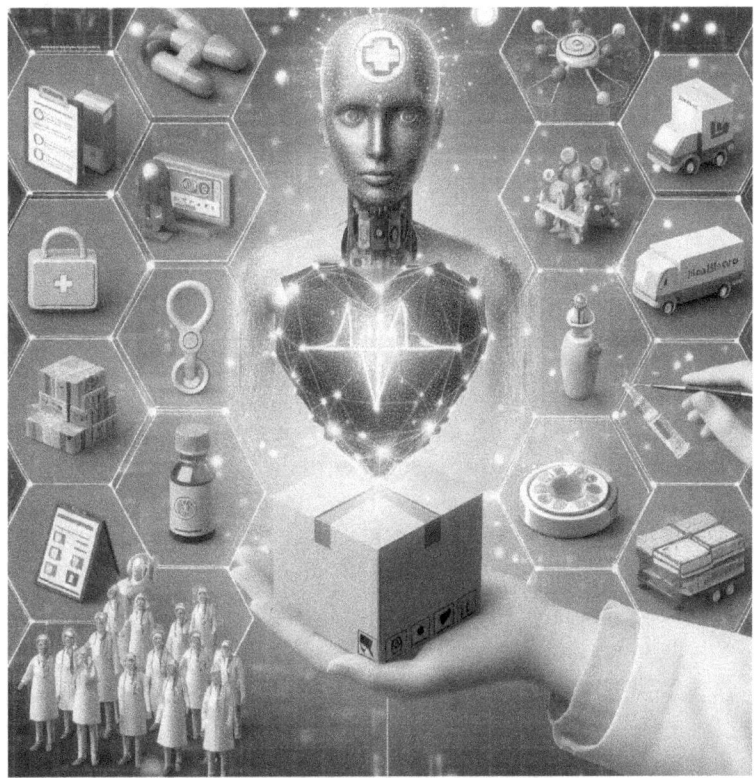

Here's an in-depth exploration of why AI adoption in healthcare operations and management is crucial:

1. **Enhanced Decision-making in Healthcare Delivery:** AI enables healthcare organizations to make data-driven decisions by analyzing extensive datasets from electronic health records (EHRs), medical imaging, patient monitoring devices, and administrative systems. AI algorithms can identify patterns in patient data, predict

disease progression, and recommend personalized treatment plans. This capability enhances clinical decision-making accuracy, supports evidence-based practices, and improves patient outcomes.

2. **Process Automation and Efficiency:** AI-powered automation streamlines administrative tasks, such as appointment scheduling, billing, and inventory management, reducing administrative burden and operational costs. Machine learning algorithms optimize resource allocation, streamline workflow processes, and improve hospital bed management, enhancing operational efficiency and patient flow. Automated systems also ensure compliance with regulatory standards and healthcare protocols.

3. **Improved Patient Experience and Personalized Care:** AI technologies enhance patient engagement and satisfaction by personalizing healthcare experiences. Natural language processing (NLP) and sentiment analysis analyze patient feedback, enabling healthcare providers to respond promptly to patient inquiries and concerns. AI-driven virtual assistants provide personalized health recommendations, medication reminders, and lifestyle advice, fostering patient adherence to treatment plans and promoting wellness.

4. **Enhanced Productivity and Innovation:** AI tools augment healthcare professionals' productivity by automating routine tasks, such as medical transcription, data entry, and diagnostic image analysis. AI-powered diagnostic systems analyze medical images, detect anomalies, and assist radiologists in interpreting results accurately. This frees up healthcare professionals to focus on complex clinical tasks, research initiatives, and innovative healthcare solutions.

5. **Predictive Analytics and Insights:** AI enables predictive analytics to forecast healthcare trends, patient outcomes, and population health metrics. By analyzing historical patient data and epidemiological trends, AI algorithms

identify high-risk patient populations, anticipate disease outbreaks, and optimize preventive care strategies. Predictive analytics support proactive intervention, resource allocation, and healthcare planning, enhancing operational preparedness and public health initiatives.

6. **Competitive Advantage in Healthcare Delivery:** Organizations leveraging AI gain a competitive edge by optimizing healthcare delivery processes, reducing treatment costs, and improving patient satisfaction metrics. AI-driven innovations in telemedicine, remote patient monitoring, and personalized medicine attract patients seeking convenient, high-quality healthcare services. By integrating AI technologies, healthcare providers differentiate themselves in a competitive marketplace and maintain leadership in patient-centered care.

7. **Scalability and Cost Savings:** Cloud-based AI platforms facilitate scalable healthcare solutions, enabling seamless integration of patient data, medical records, and diagnostic insights across healthcare networks. AI technologies support scalable telehealth services, virtual consultations, and remote patient monitoring programs, expanding access to healthcare services while reducing operational overhead. AI-driven efficiencies minimize healthcare expenditures, optimize resource utilization, and support sustainable healthcare delivery models.

8. **Risk Mitigation and Compliance:** AI enhances healthcare compliance by automating regulatory reporting, monitoring patient data privacy, and detecting potential security breaches. AI-powered systems analyze healthcare data for anomalies, ensuring adherence to data protection regulations (e.g., HIPAA) and mitigating cybersecurity risks. Proactive risk management strategies safeguard patient confidentiality, uphold regulatory standards, and maintain trust in healthcare operations.

In summary, AI adoption in healthcare operations and management empowers organizations to optimize clinical workflows, enhance patient care delivery, and drive healthcare innovation. By leveraging AI technologies, healthcare providers improve decision-making processes, automate administrative tasks, and deliver personalized healthcare experiences that prioritize patient outcomes and operational excellence. Embracing AI enables healthcare organizations to navigate complex healthcare challenges, improve healthcare access, and achieve sustainable growth in the evolving healthcare landscape.

Examples:

1. **Enhanced Decision-making in Healthcare Delivery:**

   Company/Software: Optum, GE Healthcare

   Example: Optum uses AI-powered analytics to optimize healthcare delivery decisions. Their platform integrates clinical and operational data to improve resource allocation, enhance patient flow management, and reduce wait times, thereby optimizing healthcare delivery in hospitals and clinics.

2. **Process Automation and Efficiency:**

   Company/Software: LeanTaaS, Olive AI

   Example: Olive AI automates administrative tasks in healthcare operations using AI-driven robotic process automation (RPA). Their platform streamlines scheduling, billing, and administrative workflows, improving efficiency and reducing operational costs across healthcare organizations.

3. **Improved Patient Experience and Personalized Care:**

   Company/Software: Cerner, PatientMatters

   Example: Cerner employs AI to personalize patient experiences in healthcare settings. Their platform analyzes patient data to provide personalized treatment recommendations, enhance communication between patients and providers, and improve overall patient satisfaction and outcomes.

4. **Enhanced Productivity and Innovation:**

   > **Company/Software: IBM Watson Health, Innovaccer**
   >
   > **Example:** IBM Watson Health integrates AI to drive productivity and innovation in healthcare operations. Their platform applies AI algorithms for population health management, predictive analytics for disease prevention, and fostering innovation in medical research and healthcare delivery.

5. **Predictive Analytics and Insights:**

   > **Company/Software: SyTrue, Apixio**
   >
   > **Example:** Apixio uses AI-driven predictive analytics to derive insights from unstructured healthcare data. Their platform applies natural language processing (NLP) and machine learning to identify patterns in patient records, predict health outcomes, and inform clinical decision-making for improved patient care.

6. **Competitive Advantage in Healthcare Delivery:**

   > **Company/Software: Siemens Healthineers, Innovaccer**
   >
   > **Example:** Innovaccer leverages AI to provide a competitive advantage in healthcare delivery. Their platform integrates data from disparate sources to create comprehensive patient profiles, optimize care coordination, and differentiate healthcare providers through improved operational efficiency and patient outcomes.

7. **Scalability and Cost Savings:**

   > **Company/Software: Tempus, Pieces Technologies**
   >
   > **Example:** Tempus applies AI to scale healthcare operations and achieve cost savings. Their platform uses machine learning for precision medicine, optimizing clinical workflows, and reducing healthcare costs through efficient resource allocation and patient management strategies.

8. **Risk Mitigation and Compliance:**

> **Company/Software: Nuance Communications, Health Catalyst**
>
> **Example:** Health Catalyst uses AI to mitigate risks and ensure compliance in healthcare operations. Their platform applies AI-driven analytics to monitor quality metrics, detect anomalies in healthcare data, and maintain regulatory compliance, thereby enhancing patient safety and data security.

These examples demonstrate how AI technologies are transforming healthcare operations and management by enhancing decision-making, automating processes, improving patient care experiences, driving productivity and innovation, and ensuring compliance with regulatory standards.

6.1 AI in Healthcare Supply Chain Management

Artificial Intelligence (AI) is revolutionizing healthcare supply chain management, offering significant benefits that enhance efficiency, optimize logistics, and ensure patient-centric care delivery.

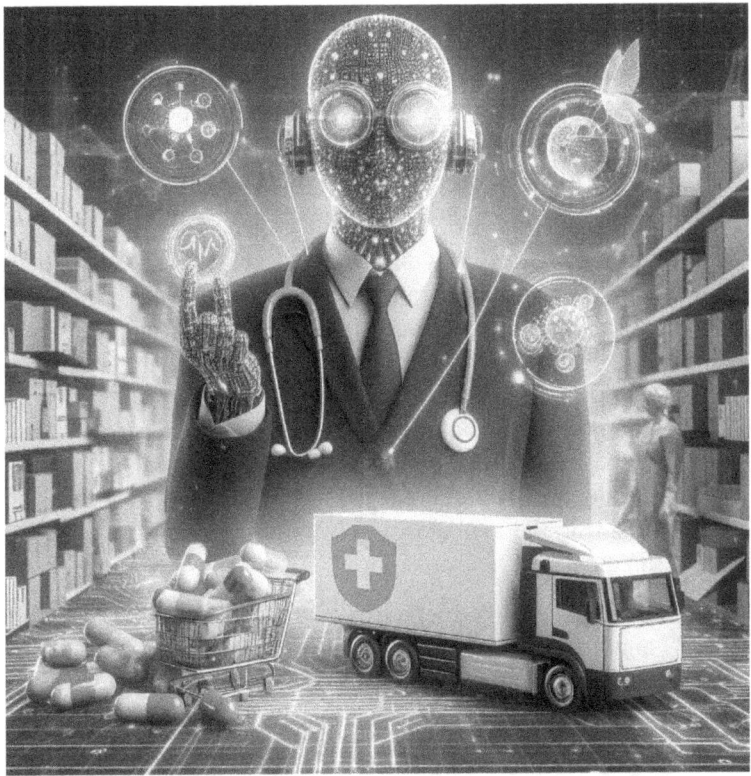

Here's an in-depth exploration of why AI adoption in healthcare supply chain management is crucial:

1. **Enhanced Decision-making and Inventory Management:** AI empowers healthcare providers to make data-driven decisions by analyzing extensive data sets related to supply chain operations. AI algorithms can predict demand patterns, optimize inventory levels, and forecast supply needs based on real-time data analytics.

This capability ensures hospitals maintain adequate stock levels of critical medical supplies and pharmaceuticals, minimizing stockouts, reducing waste, and improving resource allocation.

2. **Process Automation and Operational Efficiency:** AI-powered automation streamlines complex supply chain processes, such as procurement, distribution, and inventory management. AI algorithms automate routine tasks like order processing, vendor management, and logistics tracking, freeing up healthcare staff to focus on patient care and strategic initiatives. Automation reduces administrative burdens, enhances operational efficiency, and accelerates the supply chain cycle times, ultimately lowering operational costs.

3. **Improved Patient Care and Safety:** AI enhances patient care by ensuring timely access to essential medical supplies and pharmaceuticals. Predictive analytics and machine learning algorithms optimize supply chain workflows, enabling hospitals to respond swiftly to patient needs and emergencies. AI-driven supply chain management minimizes medication errors, enhances medication adherence, and improves patient safety by ensuring the availability of quality-assured products and medical devices.

4. **Enhanced Productivity and Innovation:** AI tools augment healthcare supply chain productivity by optimizing route planning, warehouse operations, and distribution logistics. AI-driven predictive maintenance prevents equipment breakdowns, reduces downtime, and prolongs the lifespan of medical devices and infrastructure. By automating labor-intensive tasks and leveraging AI-powered insights, healthcare supply chain managers can innovate processes, drive continuous improvement, and enhance service delivery efficiency.

5. **Predictive Analytics and Demand Forecasting:** AI enables healthcare providers to leverage predictive analytics for accurate demand forecasting and inventory

optimization. By analyzing historical data and healthcare trends, AI algorithms anticipate fluctuating demand patterns, seasonal variations, and supply chain disruptions. Predictive analytics empower supply chain managers to proactively address supply shortages, mitigate risks, and implement contingency plans to ensure uninterrupted patient care delivery.

6. **Competitive Advantage and Market Leadership:** Hospitals adopting AI-driven supply chain management gain a competitive edge by improving operational resilience, reducing costs, and enhancing service quality. AI enables healthcare providers to optimize procurement strategies, negotiate favorable contracts with suppliers, and maintain competitive pricing for medical products and services. By leveraging AI for supply chain innovation, hospitals can differentiate themselves in a competitive healthcare marketplace and strengthen their reputation for operational excellence.

7. **Scalability and Cost Savings:** AI technologies facilitate scalable supply chain solutions that accommodate expanding healthcare needs, geographical expansion, and evolving regulatory requirements. Cloud-based AI platforms centralize supply chain data, facilitate real-time collaboration with suppliers, and optimize distribution networks across multiple hospital sites. AI-driven scalability reduces procurement lead times, minimizes overhead costs, and enables hospitals to achieve cost efficiencies while maintaining service quality and patient satisfaction.

8. **Risk Mitigation and Compliance:** AI enhances healthcare supply chain compliance by automating regulatory reporting, ensuring product traceability, and monitoring supplier adherence to quality standards. AI-powered analytics detect anomalies in supply chain data, mitigate counterfeit product risks, and enhance transparency in product sourcing and distribution. Proactive risk management strategies safeguard patient safety, uphold regulatory compliance, and protect

hospitals from reputational risks associated with supply chain disruptions.

In summary, AI adoption in healthcare supply chain management optimizes logistics operations, enhances patient care quality, and drives innovation in healthcare delivery. By harnessing AI technologies, hospitals can make informed decisions, automate supply chain processes, and improve operational efficiencies that ultimately support sustainable growth and resilience in an increasingly complex healthcare environment. Embracing AI enables healthcare providers to achieve supply chain excellence, deliver value-based care, and enhance overall patient outcomes.

Examples:

1. **Enhanced Decision-making and Inventory Management:**

   Company/Software: Omnicell, Oracle Health Sciences

   Example: Omnicell uses AI-driven analytics to optimize inventory management in healthcare supply chains. Their platform integrates real-time data from hospitals and suppliers to forecast demand, reduce stockouts, and streamline inventory levels, thereby enhancing decision-making in healthcare logistics.

2. **Process Automation and Operational Efficiency:**

   Company/Software: Kinaxis, Infor Healthcare

   Example: Kinaxis leverages AI for process automation and operational efficiency in healthcare supply chain management. Their platform automates workflows, improves supply chain visibility, and optimizes inventory replenishment processes, leading to reduced costs and enhanced operational efficiency across healthcare organizations.

3. **Improved Patient Care and Safety:**

   Company/Software: BD (Becton Dickinson), GHX (Global Healthcare Exchange)

Example: BD integrates AI into healthcare supply chain management to improve patient care and safety. Their platform ensures accurate and timely delivery of medical supplies, reduces the risk of stockouts for critical items, and enhances patient safety through effective inventory management practices.

4. **Enhanced Productivity and Innovation:**

Company/Software: Vizient, SAP Healthcare

Example: Vizient applies AI to drive productivity and innovation in healthcare supply chain operations. Their platform optimizes procurement processes, fosters collaboration between healthcare providers and suppliers, and promotes innovation in supply chain logistics to meet the evolving needs of healthcare delivery.

5. **Predictive Analytics and Demand Forecasting:**

Company/Software: Syft Analytics, Apervita

Example: Syft Analytics uses AI-powered predictive analytics for demand forecasting in healthcare supply chain management. Their platform analyzes historical data, patient trends, and clinical insights to forecast demand for medical supplies, optimize inventory levels, and improve supply chain resilience and responsiveness.

6. **Competitive Advantage and Market Leadership:**

Company/Software: Premier Inc., IBM Watson Health

Example: Premier Inc. leverages AI to achieve competitive advantage in healthcare supply chain management. Their platform integrates AI-driven analytics to optimize procurement strategies, reduce costs, and enhance supply chain agility, positioning healthcare providers for market leadership through efficient supply chain operations.

7. **Scalability and Cost Savings:**

Company/Software: Tracelink, Omnicell

> **Example:** Tracelink employs AI for scalability and cost savings in healthcare supply chain management. Their platform utilizes AI algorithms for supply chain visibility, serialization, and compliance, enabling healthcare organizations to scale operations efficiently while reducing costs associated with inventory management and regulatory compliance.

8. **Risk Mitigation and Compliance:**

   > **Company/Software: GHX (Global Healthcare Exchange), Veeva Systems**
   >
   > **Example:** GHX uses AI to mitigate risks and ensure compliance in healthcare supply chain operations. Their platform monitors supplier performance, analyzes data for regulatory compliance, and enhances supply chain transparency to mitigate risks associated with product recalls, shortages, and regulatory changes.

These examples illustrate how AI technologies are transforming healthcare supply chain management by improving decision-making, automating processes, enhancing patient care and safety, driving productivity and innovation, predicting demand, ensuring competitive advantage, achieving scalability and cost savings, and mitigating risks through compliance measures.

6.2 AI for Workforce Management and Scheduling

Artificial Intelligence (AI) is playing a pivotal role in transforming workforce management and scheduling practices within the healthcare industry. The application of AI technologies offers substantial benefits, ranging from optimizing staff allocation to enhancing patient care delivery.

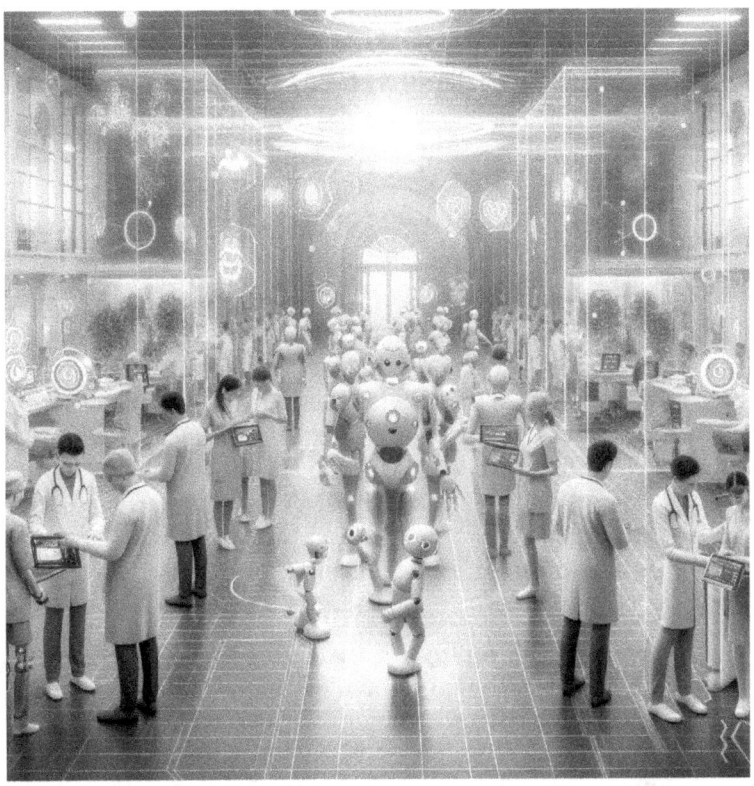

Here's a detailed exploration of why AI adoption in workforce management and scheduling is crucial for healthcare organizations:

1. **Enhanced Staffing Optimization through Predictive Analytics:** AI enables healthcare facilities to optimize staffing levels based on predictive analytics. By analyzing historical patient data, seasonal trends, and real-time

patient influx, AI algorithms can forecast patient volumes and acuity levels. This predictive capability helps healthcare managers to adjust staffing requirements proactively, ensuring adequate coverage during peak periods and optimizing resource allocation based on anticipated demand.

2. **Automated and Efficient Scheduling:** AI-driven scheduling tools automate the complex task of creating efficient and compliant schedules for healthcare professionals. These tools consider factors such as staff availability, skills, certifications, patient needs, and regulatory requirements (like nurse-to-patient ratios). AI algorithms can generate optimized schedules that minimize overtime costs, reduce staff burnout, and ensure that the right healthcare professionals are available at the right times and locations within the facility.

3. **Improving Patient Care and Safety:** Effective workforce management facilitated by AI enhances patient care and safety by ensuring that healthcare facilities are adequately staffed with qualified professionals. AI algorithms can predict potential staffing shortages or scheduling conflicts that may impact patient care delivery. By optimizing schedules and staffing levels, healthcare organizations can mitigate risks, improve response times, and maintain high standards of patient care across different departments and shifts.

4. **Enhancing Employee Satisfaction and Retention:** AI-powered scheduling promotes employee satisfaction by allowing healthcare professionals to have more control over their schedules. AI algorithms consider staff preferences, such as shift preferences, time-off requests, and work-life balance considerations. By prioritizing these preferences and reducing instances of last-minute schedule changes, AI helps improve job satisfaction, reduce turnover rates, and enhance overall employee retention within healthcare organizations.

5. **Operational Efficiency and Cost Reduction:** AI-driven workforce management tools help healthcare organizations achieve operational efficiencies and cost savings by optimizing labor utilization. AI algorithms analyze historical data to identify staffing patterns, streamline workflow processes, and reduce unnecessary overtime expenses. By optimizing resource allocation and improving staff productivity, healthcare facilities can achieve significant cost reductions while maintaining high-quality patient care.

6. **Compliance with Regulatory Requirements:** AI enhances compliance with regulatory standards and labor laws in healthcare settings by automating scheduling practices that adhere to legal requirements. AI algorithms monitor and enforce compliance with nurse-to-patient ratios, break time regulations, and overtime limits. By ensuring adherence to these regulations, healthcare organizations minimize legal risks, avoid penalties, and uphold ethical standards in workforce management practices.

7. **Continuous Learning and Adaptability:** AI-driven workforce management solutions continuously learn from data patterns and employee feedback to refine scheduling algorithms and improve operational outcomes over time. By analyzing performance metrics and adjusting scheduling strategies based on real-time data, AI helps healthcare facilities adapt to changing patient needs, staff preferences, and organizational priorities. This adaptability enables healthcare organizations to respond effectively to dynamic healthcare environments and maintain operational agility.

8. **Integration with Healthcare Systems:** AI integrates seamlessly with electronic health records (EHRs), payroll systems, and other healthcare IT infrastructure to create a cohesive workforce management ecosystem. Integrated AI platforms facilitate real-time data exchange, synchronize scheduling with patient appointments, and provide comprehensive analytics for strategic decision-

making. This integration promotes efficiency, enhances communication between departments, and supports holistic workforce management strategies aligned with healthcare delivery goals.

In summary, AI adoption in workforce management and scheduling is essential for healthcare organizations to optimize staffing, improve patient care delivery, and enhance employee satisfaction. By leveraging AI-driven predictive analytics, automation, and compliance tools, healthcare facilities can achieve operational excellence, reduce costs, and maintain high standards of care. Embracing AI enables healthcare organizations to navigate staffing challenges effectively, promote workforce well-being, and uphold patient safety in a rapidly evolving healthcare landscape.

Examples:

1. **Enhanced Staffing Optimization through Predictive Analytics:**

Company/Software: Kronos Incorporated, Allocate Software
Example: Allocate Software utilizes AI-driven predictive analytics for workforce management in healthcare. Their platform analyzes historical data, patient admission rates, and seasonal trends to optimize staffing levels, ensuring the right mix of healthcare professionals are available to meet patient demand efficiently.

2. **Automated and Efficient Scheduling:**

Company/Software: ShiftWizard, AMiON
Example: ShiftWizard employs AI to automate and optimize scheduling in healthcare settings. Their platform uses AI algorithms to create schedules based on staff availability, patient needs, and workload forecasts, improving efficiency and reducing scheduling conflicts among healthcare professionals.

3. **Improving Patient Care and Safety:**

> **Company/Software: Cerner Corporation, Q-nomy**
>
> **Example:** Cerner Corporation integrates AI into workforce management to improve patient care and safety. Their platform optimizes scheduling to ensure adequate staffing levels in critical care areas, minimizes wait times, and enhances patient flow management for better clinical outcomes and patient safety.

4. **Enhancing Employee Satisfaction and Retention:**

> **Company/Software: HealthcareSource, OnShift**
>
> **Example:** OnShift utilizes AI to enhance employee satisfaction and retention in healthcare workforce management. Their platform considers staff preferences, workload balance, and skill matching to create schedules that align with employee needs, fostering a positive work environment and reducing turnover rates.

5. **Operational Efficiency and Cost Reduction:**

> **Company/Software: Syft (by Indeed), SmartLinx Solutions**
>
> **Example:** SmartLinx Solutions applies AI for workforce management in healthcare to enhance operational efficiency and reduce costs. Their platform optimizes labor allocation, improves resource utilization, and streamlines scheduling processes, leading to cost savings and improved financial performance for healthcare organizations.

6. **Compliance with Regulatory Requirements:**

> **Company/Software: API Healthcare (a GE Healthcare Company), BambooHR**
>
> **Example**: API Healthcare integrates AI into workforce management to ensure compliance with regulatory requirements in healthcare settings. Their platform automates scheduling practices that align with labor laws, union agreements, and accreditation standards, minimizing compliance risks and penalties.

7. **Continuous Learning and Adaptability:**

Company/Software: Vizient, Saviynt
Example: Vizient uses AI for continuous learning and adaptability in healthcare workforce management. Their platform analyzes scheduling patterns, staff performance data, and patient outcomes to continuously improve scheduling algorithms and adapt to changing healthcare demands effectively.

8. **Integration with Healthcare Systems:**

Company/Software: Allscripts, Meditech
Example: Allscripts leverages AI to integrate workforce management and scheduling seamlessly with healthcare systems. Their platform ensures interoperability between scheduling software and electronic health records (EHRs), facilitating real-time data exchange for better decision-making and operational efficiency in healthcare facilities.

These examples demonstrate how AI technologies are transforming workforce management and scheduling in healthcare by optimizing staffing, improving operational efficiency, enhancing patient care and safety, boosting employee satisfaction, ensuring regulatory compliance, fostering continuous learning, and integrating seamlessly with existing healthcare systems.

6.3 AI in Healthcare warehouse and storage management

Artificial Intelligence (AI) is revolutionizing healthcare warehouse and storage management by enhancing operational efficiency, optimizing inventory control, and ensuring compliance with regulatory standards.

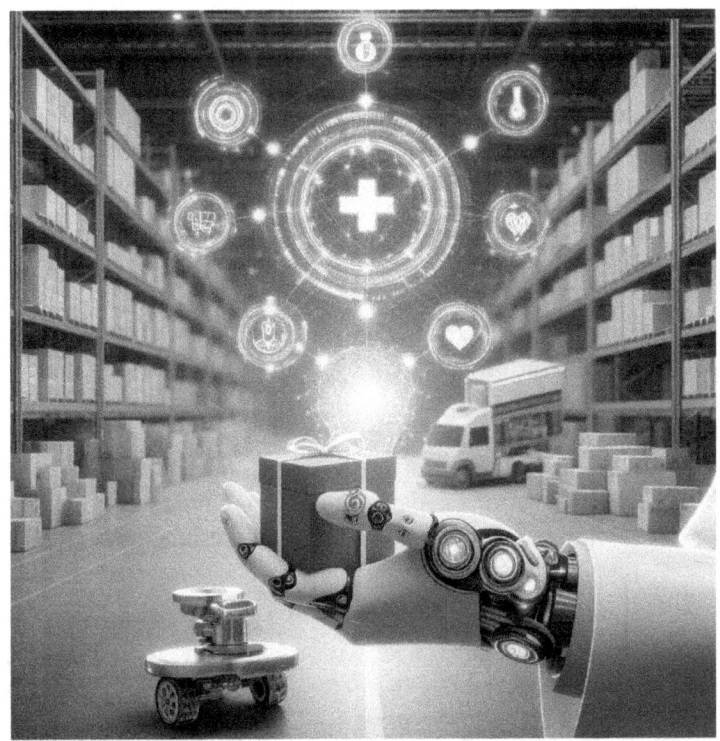

Here are key reasons why AI adoption in this area is crucial:

1. **Enhanced Inventory Management:** AI enables healthcare facilities to manage inventory effectively by analyzing consumption patterns, predicting demand fluctuations, and optimizing stock levels. AI algorithms can track perishable items, monitor expiration dates, and automate replenishment processes, ensuring adequate supply availability while minimizing wastage.

2. **Process Automation and Efficiency:** AI-powered automation streamlines warehouse operations by automating routine tasks such as inventory counting, order picking, and storage optimization. Robotic systems equipped with AI algorithms can navigate warehouse environments autonomously, accelerate order fulfillment, and reduce operational costs associated with manual labor.

3. **Temperature and Environment Monitoring:** AI technologies monitor environmental conditions within healthcare warehouses to ensure optimal storage conditions for sensitive pharmaceuticals, vaccines, and medical supplies. AI-powered sensors detect deviations in temperature, humidity levels, and light exposure, triggering real-time alerts to prevent product degradation and maintain quality standards.

4. **Predictive Maintenance and Equipment Optimization:** AI-driven predictive analytics anticipate equipment failures, schedule maintenance activities proactively, and optimize the performance of warehouse machinery. Machine learning algorithms analyze equipment sensor data, predict maintenance needs, and minimize downtime, enhancing operational reliability and reducing maintenance costs.

5. **Regulatory Compliance and Quality Assurance:** AI facilitates compliance with regulatory guidelines and quality assurance standards in healthcare warehouse management. AI-powered systems audit storage conditions, track product traceability, and ensure adherence to Good Distribution Practices (GDP) and Good Manufacturing Practices (GMP), safeguarding product integrity and patient safety.

6. **Data-driven Decision-making:** AI empowers healthcare providers to make data-driven decisions by analyzing warehouse performance metrics, inventory turnover rates, and supply chain efficiency. AI algorithms identify operational bottlenecks, optimize workflow processes,

and support strategic planning initiatives to enhance warehouse productivity and operational resilience.

7. **Cost Savings and Resource Optimization:** AI technologies optimize resource allocation, reduce inventory holding costs, and minimize supply chain inefficiencies in healthcare warehouse management. AI-driven demand forecasting models anticipate procurement needs, optimize storage space utilization, and streamline logistics operations, achieving cost savings and improving financial sustainability.

8. **Security and Risk Management:** AI enhances security measures in healthcare warehouses by detecting anomalies, monitoring access control, and preventing unauthorized entry. AI-powered surveillance systems analyze video feeds, identify suspicious activities, and mitigate risks related to theft, product tampering, and inventory shrinkage, safeguarding valuable assets and ensuring regulatory compliance.

In summary, AI adoption in healthcare warehouse and storage management is essential for optimizing inventory control, enhancing operational efficiency, and ensuring regulatory compliance. By leveraging AI technologies in inventory management, process automation, and predictive analytics, healthcare organizations can achieve cost savings, improve patient care delivery, and maintain high standards of operational excellence in warehouse operations.

Examples:

1. **Enhanced Inventory Management:**

Company/Software: Cardinal Health, Omnicell
Example: Cardinal Health uses AI to enhance inventory management in healthcare warehouses. Their system integrates AI algorithms to predict demand for medical supplies, optimize stock levels, and reduce wastage, ensuring critical supplies are available when needed across hospital networks.

2. **Process Automation and Efficiency:**

> **Company/Software: Swisslog Healthcare, BD Pyxis**
>
> **Example:** Swisslog Healthcare leverages AI for process automation and efficiency in healthcare warehouse management. Their AI-powered systems automate inventory replenishment, track item usage patterns, and optimize storage layout, improving operational efficiency and reducing manual handling errors.

3. **Temperature and Environment Monitoring:**

> **Company/Software: Temptime Corporation, SensiTech**
>
> **Example:** Temptime Corporation integrates AI for temperature and environment monitoring in healthcare storage facilities. Their AI systems continuously monitor temperature-sensitive medical supplies, alerting staff to deviations and ensuring compliance with regulatory requirements for storing medications and vaccines.

4. **Predictive Maintenance and Equipment Optimization:**

> **Company/Software: Siemens Healthineers, GE Healthcare**
>
> **Example:** Siemens Healthineers applies AI for predictive maintenance and equipment optimization in healthcare warehouse management. Their AI solutions analyze equipment performance data, predict maintenance needs, and optimize asset utilization, reducing downtime and ensuring reliable operation of storage and retrieval systems.

5. **Regulatory Compliance and Quality Assurance:**

> **Company/Software: TraceLink, DHL Life Sciences & Healthcare**
>
> **Example:** TraceLink uses AI for regulatory compliance and quality assurance in healthcare warehouse management. Their AI-driven platform ensures traceability of pharmaceuticals, tracks product serialization, and verifies compliance with regulatory standards such as FDA and EU guidelines for drug storage and distribution.

6. **Data-driven Decision-making:**

> **Company/Software: Omnicell, McKesson Corporation**
>
> **Example:** Omnicell employs AI for data-driven decision-making in healthcare warehouse management. Their AI systems analyze historical data, patient demand patterns, and inventory turnover rates to optimize procurement decisions, improve supply chain efficiency, and enhance patient care outcomes.

7. **Cost Savings and Resource Optimization:**

> **Company/Software: Oracle Health Sciences, CliniSys Group**
>
> **Example:** Oracle Health Sciences utilizes AI for cost savings and resource optimization in healthcare warehouse management. Their AI solutions optimize inventory levels, streamline procurement processes, and minimize excess stock, reducing costs associated with storage, handling, and procurement of medical supplies.

8. **Security and Risk Management:**

> **Company/Software: Johnson Controls, Tyco Integrated Security**
>
> **Example:** Johnson Controls integrates AI for security and risk management in healthcare warehouse facilities. Their AI-powered security systems monitor access control, detect anomalies in storage areas, and ensure compliance with HIPAA regulations, safeguarding sensitive medical supplies and protecting against theft or tampering.

These examples illustrate how AI technologies are transforming healthcare warehouse and storage management by enhancing inventory management, automating processes, monitoring environmental conditions, predicting maintenance needs, ensuring regulatory compliance, enabling data-driven decision-making, optimizing resources, and improving security and risk management.

7. AI in Genomics and Bioinformatics

Artificial Intelligence (AI) is revolutionizing genomics and bioinformatics in healthcare, offering transformative capabilities that enhance research, diagnosis, and personalized treatment. The adoption of AI in this field is crucial due to its potential to drive innovation, improve decision-making, and advance competitiveness.

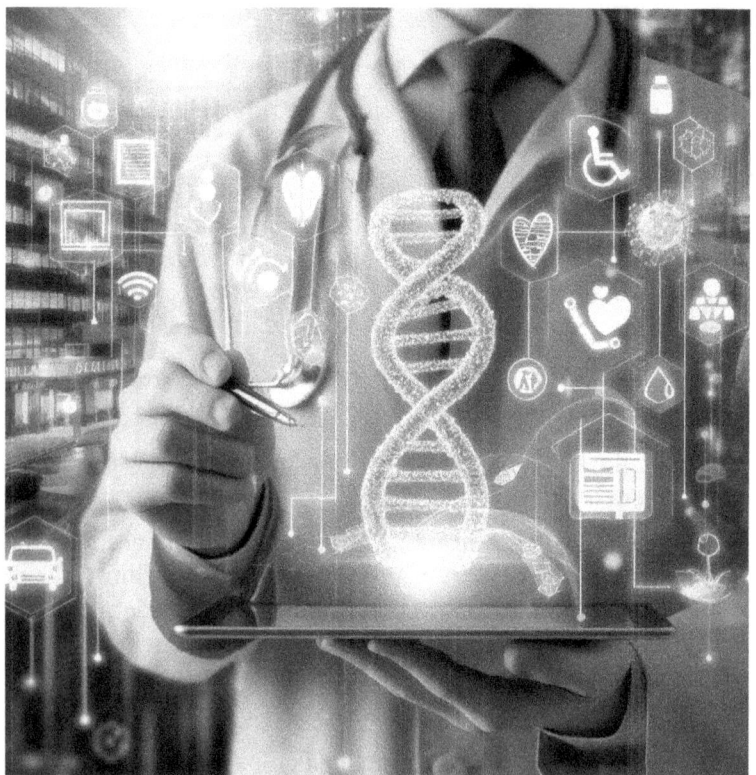

Here's a detailed exploration of why AI adoption in genomics and bioinformatics is essential:

1. **Enhanced Data Analysis and Interpretation:** AI enables healthcare professionals and researchers to analyze vast amounts of genomic data efficiently. AI algorithms can process complex genomic sequences, identify patterns, and detect variations that may indicate

genetic predispositions to diseases or potential treatment responses. By analyzing both structured genomic data (such as DNA sequences) and unstructured data (such as medical literature), AI enhances the accuracy and speed of genomic analysis, leading to more precise diagnostics and treatment strategies.

2. **Accelerated Drug Discovery and Development:** AI-powered bioinformatics tools accelerate drug discovery processes by predicting drug-target interactions, identifying biomarkers, and optimizing therapeutic compounds. AI algorithms can analyze genomic data to pinpoint molecular targets for new drugs or repurpose existing drugs for different indications. This capability reduces research and development timelines, lowers costs, and facilitates the discovery of innovative treatments tailored to genetic profiles and disease subtypes.

3. **Personalized Medicine and Treatment Optimization:** AI in genomics enables personalized medicine approaches by integrating genomic data with clinical information. AI algorithms analyze patient-specific genomic profiles to predict disease risks, select optimal treatment regimens, and customize dosages based on genetic factors. This personalized approach improves treatment outcomes, minimizes adverse effects, and enhances patient adherence to therapies tailored to their genetic makeup.

4. **Predictive Analytics for Disease Prevention and Early Detection:** AI-driven predictive analytics leverage genomic data to forecast disease risks, detect genetic predispositions, and enable early intervention strategies. AI algorithms analyze genetic markers associated with diseases to identify high-risk individuals who may benefit from targeted screening programs or preventive measures. By predicting disease trajectories and outcomes, AI supports proactive healthcare interventions aimed at reducing disease burden and improving population health.

5. **Facilitation of Precision Diagnostics and Prognostics:** AI enhances diagnostic accuracy in healthcare by interpreting genomic data to diagnose genetic disorders, characterize tumor mutations, and predict disease progression. AI algorithms can distinguish between benign and malignant genetic variations, classify disease subtypes, and stratify patients based on prognosis. This precision in diagnostics empowers clinicians to make informed decisions regarding treatment options and patient management strategies.

6. **Innovation in Bioinformatics Tools and Platforms:** AI-driven bioinformatics tools and platforms innovate research methodologies and data analysis techniques in genomics. AI algorithms continuously learn from data patterns, refine predictive models, and optimize computational workflows for genome sequencing, variant calling, and molecular modeling. This innovation fosters collaboration among researchers, accelerates scientific discoveries, and expands the application of genomics in clinical practice.

7. **Compliance with Regulatory Standards and Ethical Guidelines:** AI supports compliance with regulatory standards and ethical guidelines governing genomic data privacy, security, and informed consent. AI-powered systems ensure the responsible use of genomic data by implementing robust data governance frameworks, anonymizing patient information, and adhering to regulatory requirements for genomic research and clinical trials. By safeguarding patient confidentiality and upholding ethical standards, AI promotes trust in genomic technologies and enhances healthcare transparency.

8. **Empowering Healthcare Providers and Researchers:** AI empowers healthcare providers and researchers with actionable insights derived from complex genomic datasets. AI-driven decision support systems integrate genomic findings with clinical knowledge to inform treatment decisions, predict treatment responses, and monitor disease progression. By augmenting human

expertise with AI-driven analytics, healthcare professionals can deliver patient-centered care, advance scientific understanding of genetic diseases, and drive continuous improvement in genomic medicine.

In summary, AI adoption in genomics and bioinformatics is essential for healthcare organizations to leverage genomic data effectively, advance precision medicine initiatives, and accelerate scientific discoveries. By harnessing AI technologies for data analysis, drug discovery, personalized treatment planning, and predictive analytics, healthcare stakeholders can enhance patient care outcomes, optimize research efforts, and lead innovation in genomic healthcare solutions. Embracing AI-driven approaches in genomics enables organizations to navigate complexities, achieve operational excellence, and unlock new opportunities for improving population health and individualized patient care.

Examples:

1. **Enhanced Data Analysis and Interpretation:**

Company/Software: DNAnexus, Seven Bridges Genomics
Example: DNAnexus provides a cloud-based platform that integrates AI for enhanced data analysis and interpretation in genomics. Their AI algorithms analyze genomic data sets, identify genetic variations, and correlate them with clinical outcomes, accelerating research discoveries and personalized medicine advancements.

2. **Accelerated Drug Discovery and Development:**

Company/Software: Insilico Medicine, BenevolentAI
Example: Insilico Medicine uses AI for accelerated drug discovery and development in genomics and bioinformatics. Their AI-driven platforms predict novel drug targets, design molecular structures, and optimize drug candidates by analyzing vast datasets, significantly reducing the time and cost of bringing new therapies to market.

3. **Personalized Medicine and Treatment Optimization:**

Company/Software: Tempus Labs, SOPHiA GENETICS

Example: Tempus Labs employs AI for personalized medicine and treatment optimization using genomics data. Their AI analytics interpret genomic profiles, identify biomarkers, and generate actionable insights that guide clinicians in selecting optimal therapies tailored to individual patient genetics, improving treatment outcomes.

4. **Predictive Analytics for Disease Prevention and Early Detection:**

Company/Software: Grail, Foundation Medicine

Example: Grail utilizes AI for predictive analytics in disease prevention and early detection through genomics. Their AI algorithms analyze circulating tumor DNA to detect cancer at early stages, predict disease risks based on genetic predispositions, and enable proactive interventions for improved patient outcomes.

5. **Facilitation of Precision Diagnostics and Prognostics:**

Company/Software: Fabric Genomics, SOPHiA DDM

Example: Fabric Genomics facilitates precision diagnostics and prognostics with AI in genomics and bioinformatics. Their AI-driven clinical decision support tools interpret genomic data, provide diagnostic insights for rare diseases and genetic disorders, and predict disease progression to guide personalized patient management strategies.

6. **Innovation in Bioinformatics Tools and Platforms:**

Company/Software: Basepair, QIAGEN Bioinformatics

Example: Basepair innovates bioinformatics tools and platforms with AI in genomics. Their AI-powered software automates genomic data analysis pipelines, identifies variants, and performs functional annotations, enhancing research productivity and enabling discoveries in fields such as population genetics and microbiome studies.

7. **Compliance with Regulatory Standards and Ethical Guidelines:**

   Company/Software: Illumina, Thermo Fisher Scientific

   Example: Illumina ensures compliance with regulatory standards and ethical guidelines using AI in genomics and bioinformatics. Their AI systems monitor data privacy, ensure secure handling of genomic information, and comply with regulatory requirements such as HIPAA and GDPR, maintaining trust and ethical integrity in genomic research and clinical applications.

8. **Empowering Healthcare Providers and Researchers:**

   Company/Software: 10x Genomics, PacBio

   Example: 10x Genomics empowers healthcare providers and researchers with AI in genomics and bioinformatics. Their AI-driven solutions enable high-resolution genomic profiling, single-cell analysis, and spatial transcriptomics, facilitating new insights into disease mechanisms and accelerating scientific discoveries in precision medicine.

These examples highlight how AI technologies are transforming genomics and bioinformatics by enabling enhanced data analysis, accelerating drug discovery, facilitating personalized medicine, predicting disease risks, innovating bioinformatics tools, ensuring regulatory compliance, and empowering healthcare providers and researchers worldwide.

7.1 AI in Genetic Sequencing and Analysis

Artificial Intelligence (AI) is playing a transformative role in genetic sequencing and analysis within the healthcare industry. Its adoption is increasingly crucial due to its potential to revolutionize medical research, diagnosis, and treatment strategies.

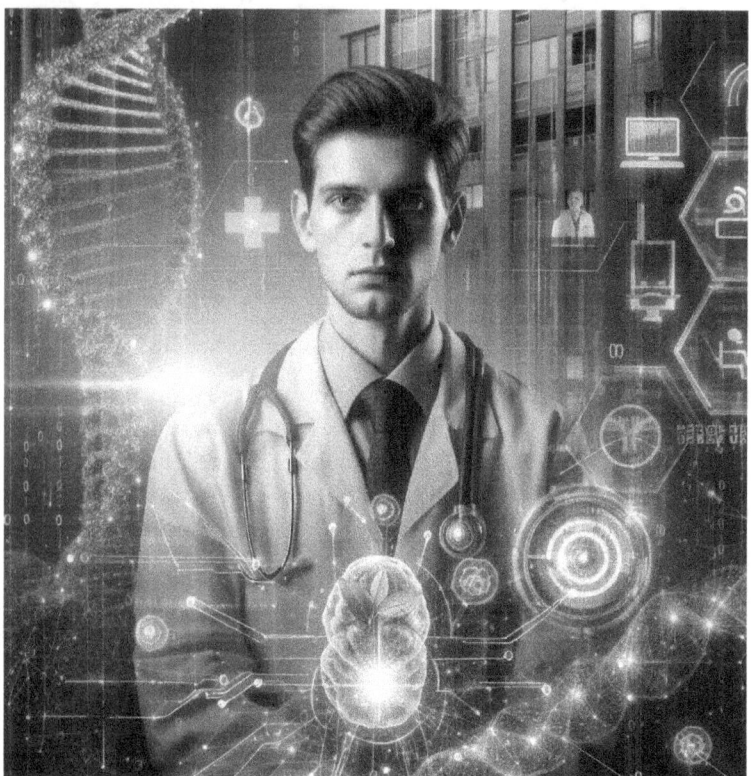

Here's an in-depth exploration of why AI adoption in genetic sequencing and analysis is essential:

1. **Enhanced Data Processing and Interpretation:** AI enables healthcare professionals and researchers to analyze vast amounts of genetic data quickly and accurately. AI algorithms excel in identifying patterns, variations, and genetic mutations within DNA sequences that may be indicative of diseases or treatment responses. By processing both structured genetic data (such as nucleotide sequences) and unstructured data (such as

medical literature and patient records), AI enhances the precision and efficiency of genetic analysis, leading to more accurate diagnostics and personalized treatment recommendations.

2. **Accelerated Genomic Research and Drug Discovery:** AI-powered tools in genetic sequencing expedite genomic research and drug discovery processes. AI algorithms can predict drug-target interactions, identify biomarkers associated with diseases, and optimize drug candidates based on genetic insights. This capability reduces the time and cost required for drug development, facilitates the discovery of targeted therapies tailored to genetic profiles, and supports the advancement of precision medicine initiatives.

3. **Personalized Medicine and Treatment Optimization:** AI in genetic sequencing enables personalized medicine by leveraging genomic data to tailor treatments to individual patients. AI algorithms analyze genetic profiles to predict disease risks, optimize treatment protocols, and anticipate patient responses to medications. This personalized approach enhances treatment efficacy, minimizes adverse effects, and improves patient outcomes by aligning therapies with genetic predispositions and disease susceptibilities.

4. **Predictive Analytics for Disease Prevention and Management:** AI-driven predictive analytics utilize genetic information to forecast disease risks, preemptively detect genetic predispositions, and guide preventive healthcare strategies. AI algorithms analyze genetic markers to identify individuals at higher risk of developing certain conditions, enabling proactive interventions such as early screening programs or lifestyle modifications. By predicting disease trajectories and outcomes, AI supports preventive healthcare efforts aimed at reducing disease incidence and improving population health outcomes.

5. **Innovation in Bioinformatics and Computational Genomics:** AI fosters innovation in bioinformatics and computational genomics by enhancing data analysis techniques and computational modeling. AI algorithms continuously learn from genomic datasets, refine predictive models, and optimize workflows for genome sequencing, variant calling, and molecular profiling. This innovation accelerates scientific discoveries, expands the application of genomics in clinical practice, and facilitates collaborative research efforts among scientists and healthcare providers.

6. **Compliance with Regulatory Standards and Ethical Guidelines:** AI supports compliance with regulatory standards and ethical guidelines governing genetic data privacy, security, and informed consent. AI-powered systems ensure the responsible use of genetic information by implementing robust data governance frameworks, anonymizing patient data, and adhering to regulatory requirements for genetic research and clinical trials. By safeguarding patient confidentiality and upholding ethical standards, AI promotes trust in genomic technologies and supports transparent healthcare practices.

7. **Empowering Healthcare Providers and Researchers:** AI empowers healthcare providers and researchers with actionable insights derived from complex genetic data. AI-driven decision support systems integrate genomic findings with clinical knowledge to inform treatment decisions, predict disease progression, and guide patient management strategies. By augmenting human expertise with AI-driven analytics, healthcare professionals can deliver personalized care, advance genetic research initiatives, and improve health outcomes across diverse patient populations.

In summary, AI adoption in genetic sequencing and analysis is indispensable for healthcare organizations seeking to leverage genomic insights effectively, advance precision medicine initiatives, and pioneer innovative healthcare solutions. By harnessing AI technologies for data analysis, drug discovery, personalized treatment planning, and predictive analytics, healthcare stakeholders can optimize clinical workflows, enhance patient care outcomes, and drive continuous improvement in genomic healthcare delivery. Embracing AI-driven approaches in genetic sequencing enables organizations to navigate complexities, achieve operational excellence, and unlock new opportunities for improving public health and individualized patient care.

Examples:

1. **Enhanced Data Processing and Interpretation:**

   Company/Software: Illumina, PacBio

   Example: Illumina utilizes AI for enhanced data processing and interpretation in genetic sequencing. Their AI algorithms analyze vast genomic datasets, detect variations, and interpret genetic findings to provide insights into disease mechanisms and potential therapeutic targets, advancing personalized medicine and genomic research.

2. **Accelerated Genomic Research and Drug Discovery:**

   Company/Software: BenevolentAI, Atomwise

   Example: BenevolentAI accelerates genomic research and drug discovery using AI in genetic sequencing and analysis. Their AI-driven platforms predict novel drug targets, design molecules, and optimize drug candidates by integrating genomic data with AI algorithms, facilitating faster development of precision medicines for various diseases.

3. **Personalized Medicine and Treatment Optimization:**

   Company/Software: Tempus Labs, SOPHiA GENETICS

   Example: Tempus Labs employs AI for personalized medicine and treatment optimization through genetic sequencing and analysis. Their AI-driven platforms analyze patient genomic data, identify biomarkers, and generate actionable insights that guide clinicians in selecting tailored therapies, improving patient outcomes and treatment efficacy.

4. **Predictive Analytics for Disease Prevention and Management:**

   Company/Software: Grail, Foundation Medicine

   Example: Grail uses AI for predictive analytics in disease prevention and management via genetic sequencing and analysis. Their AI algorithms analyze circulating tumor DNA, predict disease risks based on genetic profiles, and enable early detection strategies, supporting proactive healthcare interventions and improving patient survival rates.

5. **Innovation in Bioinformatics and Computational Genomics:**

   Company/Software: Basepair, QIAGEN Bioinformatics

   Example: Basepair innovates in bioinformatics and computational genomics with AI applied to genetic sequencing and analysis. Their AI-powered platforms automate genomic data analysis pipelines, identify variants, and perform functional annotations, driving advancements in understanding genetic diseases and accelerating research discoveries.

6. **Compliance with Regulatory Standards and Ethical Guidelines:**

   Company/Software: Illumina, Thermo Fisher Scientific

   Example: Thermo Fisher Scientific ensures compliance with regulatory standards and ethical guidelines using AI in genetic sequencing and analysis. Their AI systems monitor data privacy, secure handling of genomic information, and comply with regulations such as HIPAA and GDPR, maintaining ethical integrity in genomic research and clinical applications.

7. **Empowering Healthcare Providers and Researchers:**

> **Company/Software: 10x Genomics, PacBio**
>
> **Example:** 10x Genomics empowers healthcare providers and researchers with AI in genetic sequencing and analysis. Their AI-driven solutions enable high-resolution genomic profiling, single-cell analysis, and spatial transcriptomics, facilitating new insights into disease mechanisms and accelerating scientific discoveries in precision medicine.

These examples demonstrate how AI technologies are transforming genetic sequencing and analysis in healthcare by enabling enhanced data processing, accelerating research and drug discovery, facilitating personalized medicine, predicting disease risks, innovating bioinformatics tools, ensuring regulatory compliance, and empowering healthcare providers and researchers globally.

7.2 Applications of AI in Personalized Genomics

Artificial Intelligence (AI) is revolutionizing personalized genomics in healthcare, offering profound advancements in patient care, medical research, and treatment strategies.

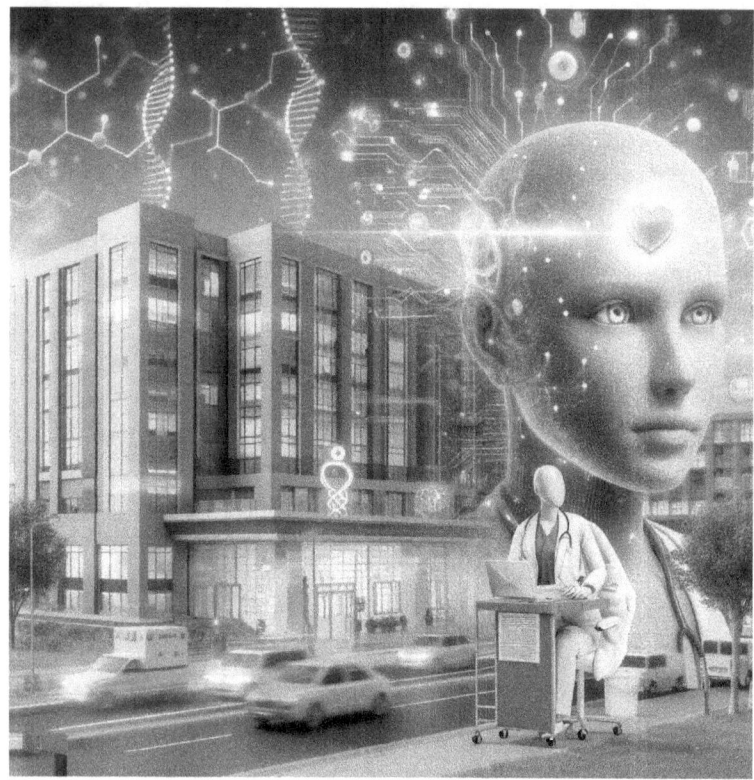

Here's an exploration of why AI adoption in personalized genomics is crucial:

1. **Enhanced Precision in Genetic Analysis:** AI empowers healthcare providers to analyze vast amounts of genetic data with unprecedented accuracy and speed. AI algorithms excel in identifying complex patterns, variations, and genetic mutations within DNA sequences, enabling precise genomic profiling of individuals. This capability enhances diagnostic accuracy, facilitates early

disease detection, and guides personalized treatment plans based on genetic predispositions and biomarkers.

2. **Facilitation of Precision Medicine Initiatives:** AI supports precision medicine by integrating genomic insights with clinical data to tailor treatments to individual patients. AI-driven platforms analyze genetic profiles to predict disease risks, optimize medication efficacy, and anticipate patient responses to therapies. This personalized approach enhances treatment outcomes, minimizes adverse effects, and fosters patient-centered care by aligning medical interventions with genetic susceptibilities and health profiles.

3. **Accelerated Drug Discovery and Development:** AI accelerates drug discovery processes by predicting drug-target interactions, identifying novel biomarkers, and optimizing therapeutic strategies based on genomic data. AI algorithms analyze genomic sequences to identify potential drug candidates, simulate molecular interactions, and expedite preclinical and clinical trials. This innovation reduces time-to-market for new therapies, enhances treatment efficacy, and addresses unmet medical needs through targeted drug development approaches.

4. **Predictive Analytics for Disease Prevention:** AI-driven predictive analytics leverage genetic information to forecast disease risks, preemptively detect genetic predispositions, and inform preventive healthcare interventions. AI algorithms analyze genetic markers to stratify populations at risk, design personalized screening programs, and implement early intervention strategies. By predicting disease trajectories and optimizing preventive measures, AI supports population health management and reduces healthcare costs associated with disease treatment.

5. **Bioinformatics Advancements and Computational Genomics:** AI fosters innovation in bioinformatics and computational genomics by enhancing data analysis

techniques and computational modeling. AI-powered platforms integrate genomic datasets, refine predictive models, and automate genome sequencing processes. This innovation facilitates collaborative research efforts, expands the scope of genomic medicine applications, and drives discoveries in disease mechanisms and genetic variability.

6. **Ethical Considerations and Regulatory Compliance:** AI ensures compliance with ethical guidelines and regulatory standards governing genetic data privacy, security, and informed consent. AI-powered systems implement robust data governance frameworks, anonymize patient information, and adhere to regulatory requirements for genomic research and clinical practice. By safeguarding patient confidentiality and upholding ethical standards, AI promotes trust in genomic technologies and supports responsible healthcare practices.

7. **Empowering Healthcare Providers and Researchers:** AI empowers healthcare providers and researchers with actionable insights derived from comprehensive genomic analyses. AI-driven decision support systems integrate genetic findings with clinical expertise to guide informed decision-making, personalize patient care pathways, and optimize resource allocation in healthcare settings. By augmenting human intelligence with AI-driven analytics, healthcare stakeholders can deliver precision medicine, advance genomic research initiatives, and improve health outcomes across diverse patient populations.

In summary, AI adoption in personalized genomics represents a pivotal advancement in healthcare delivery, research innovation, and patient outcomes. By harnessing AI technologies for genetic analysis, precision medicine initiatives, drug discovery, and predictive analytics, healthcare organizations can achieve operational excellence, drive therapeutic advancements, and realize the full potential of genomic medicine in improving public health and individualized patient care. Embracing AI-driven approaches in personalized genomics enables organizations to navigate complexities, innovate with data-driven insights, and foster continuous improvement in genomic healthcare practices.

Examples:

1. **Enhanced Precision in Genetic Analysis:**

Company/Software: DNAnexus, Sophia Genetics
Example: Sophia Genetics utilizes AI to enhance precision in genetic analysis for personalized genomics. Their AI-driven platform interprets genomic data, identifies variants linked to diseases or drug responses, and provides clinicians with actionable insights to guide personalized treatment decisions, improving patient outcomes.

2. **Facilitation of Precision Medicine Initiatives:**

Company/Software: Tempus Labs, Foundation Medicine
Example: Tempus Labs facilitates precision medicine initiatives using AI in personalized genomics. Their AI-powered analytics platform integrates patient clinical data with genomic information to identify molecular biomarkers, stratify patient populations, and recommend targeted therapies, advancing personalized treatment strategies for cancer and other diseases.

3. **Accelerated Drug Discovery and Development:**

Company/Software: BenevolentAI, Atomwise
Example: BenevolentAI accelerates drug discovery and development with AI in personalized genomics. Their AI-driven platforms predict novel drug targets, design molecules, and optimize drug candidates by leveraging genomic data, leading to faster development of precision medicines tailored to individual genetic profiles.

4. **Predictive Analytics for Disease Prevention:**

Company/Software: 23andMe, Color Genomics

Example: 23andMe applies predictive analytics using AI in personalized genomics for disease prevention. Their AI algorithms analyze genetic predispositions, lifestyle factors, and environmental influences to predict disease risks, empowering individuals to take proactive health measures and enabling early intervention strategies.

5. **Bioinformatics Advancements and Computational Genomics:**

Company/Software: Basepair, QIAGEN Bioinformatics

Example: QIAGEN Bioinformatics advances bioinformatics and computational genomics with AI in personalized genomics. Their AI-driven solutions automate genomic data analysis, identify genetic variants, and integrate multi-omics data to unravel complex disease mechanisms, accelerating research discoveries and precision medicine advancements.

6. **Ethical Considerations and Regulatory Compliance:**

Company/Software: Illumina, Thermo Fisher Scientific

Example: Illumina addresses ethical considerations and regulatory compliance using AI in personalized genomics. Their AI systems ensure secure handling of genomic data, comply with HIPAA and GDPR regulations, and uphold ethical guidelines for genetic research and clinical applications, maintaining patient privacy and data integrity.

7. **Empowering Healthcare Providers and Researchers:**

Company/Software: 10x Genomics, PacBio

Example: 10x Genomics empowers healthcare providers and researchers with AI in personalized genomics. Their AI-driven technologies enable high-resolution genomic profiling, single-cell analysis, and spatial transcriptomics, providing new insights into disease biology and facilitating collaborative research efforts to advance personalized healthcare solutions.

These examples illustrate how AI technologies are transforming personalized genomics by enhancing precision in genetic analysis, facilitating precision medicine initiatives, accelerating drug discovery, enabling predictive analytics for disease prevention, advancing bioinformatics and computational genomics, addressing ethical considerations, and empowering healthcare providers and researchers globally.

7.3 AI-driven Insights in Bioinformatics

Artificial Intelligence (AI) is revolutionizing bioinformatics in healthcare, offering profound advancements in medical research, personalized medicine, and patient care.

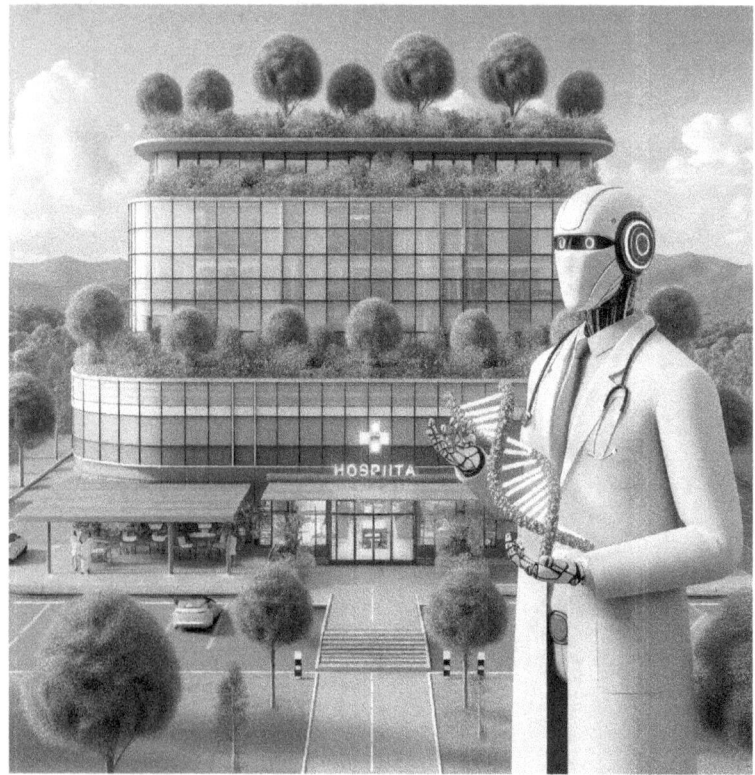

Here's an exploration of why AI adoption in bioinformatics is crucial:

1. **Enhanced Data-driven Discoveries:** AI empowers researchers and healthcare professionals to extract meaningful insights from vast datasets in bioinformatics. AI algorithms analyze genomic sequences, protein structures, and molecular interactions to uncover complex patterns and correlations. By processing large volumes of data with speed and accuracy, AI enhances the discovery of biomarkers, genetic variations, and disease

mechanisms, facilitating breakthroughs in biomedical research and drug development.

2. **Precision Medicine and Personalized Treatment:** AI supports precision medicine initiatives by integrating genomic, clinical, and lifestyle data to tailor medical treatments to individual patients. AI-driven platforms predict disease risks, optimize therapy selection, and monitor treatment responses based on genetic profiles and personalized health data. This personalized approach enhances treatment outcomes, minimizes adverse effects, and improves patient adherence to therapeutic regimens, thereby optimizing healthcare delivery and patient-centered care.

3. **Accelerated Drug Development and Design:** AI accelerates drug discovery processes by simulating molecular interactions, predicting drug-target interactions, and optimizing lead compounds based on bioinformatics data. AI algorithms analyze genomic data to identify novel drug targets, predict compound efficacy, and expedite the identification of therapeutic candidates. This innovation reduces research and development timelines, lowers costs associated with drug discovery, and expands the repertoire of targeted therapies available to patients.

4. **Predictive Analytics for Disease Prevention:** AI-powered predictive analytics utilize bioinformatics data to forecast disease risks, monitor population health trends, and implement preventive healthcare strategies. AI algorithms analyze genomic and epidemiological data to identify at-risk populations, predict disease outbreaks, and design targeted interventions for disease prevention and health promotion. By leveraging predictive models, healthcare providers can allocate resources effectively, mitigate health risks, and enhance public health outcomes across diverse populations.

5. **Bioinformatics Tools and Computational Modeling:** AI-driven bioinformatics tools advance computational

modeling and data analysis techniques essential for genomic research and clinical applications. AI platforms integrate multi-omics data, refine predictive algorithms, and automate genomic sequence analysis to expedite research workflows and improve data interpretation accuracy. This innovation facilitates collaborative research efforts, fosters interdisciplinary approaches to biomedical research, and catalyzes discoveries in disease biology and therapeutic innovation.

6. **Ethical Considerations and Regulatory Compliance:** AI ensures adherence to ethical guidelines and regulatory standards governing genomic data privacy, security, and informed consent. AI-powered systems implement robust data governance frameworks, anonymize patient information, and uphold regulatory requirements for bioinformatics research and clinical practice. By safeguarding patient confidentiality and maintaining ethical standards, AI promotes trust in genomic technologies and supports responsible healthcare practices.

7. **Empowering Healthcare Innovation and Research:** AI empowers healthcare professionals and researchers with actionable insights derived from comprehensive bioinformatics analyses. AI-driven decision support systems integrate genomic findings with clinical expertise to guide evidence-based decision-making, enhance diagnostic accuracy, and optimize treatment strategies tailored to patient-specific genetic profiles. By harnessing AI technologies, healthcare stakeholders can drive innovation in bioinformatics research, improve health outcomes, and realize the full potential of genomic medicine in transforming healthcare delivery.

In summary, AI adoption in bioinformatics represents a pivotal advancement in healthcare innovation, biomedical research, and personalized medicine. By leveraging AI-driven approaches in genomic data analysis, drug discovery, predictive analytics, and precision medicine initiatives, healthcare organizations can achieve operational excellence, drive therapeutic advancements, and enhance patient outcomes. Embracing AI technologies in bioinformatics enables organizations to navigate complexities, innovate with data-driven insights, and foster continuous improvement in genomic healthcare practices.

Examples:

1. **Enhanced Data-driven Discoveries:**

   Company/Software: DNAnexus, Seven Bridges Genomics

   Example: DNAnexus leverages AI-driven insights in bioinformatics to enhance data-driven discoveries. Their platform integrates genomic data with AI algorithms to analyze complex datasets, identify genetic variations, and uncover novel insights into disease mechanisms and treatment responses, accelerating biomedical research and precision medicine initiatives.

2. **Precision Medicine and Personalized Treatment:**

   Company/Software: Tempus Labs, SOPHiA Genetics

   Example: Tempus Labs applies AI-driven insights in bioinformatics for precision medicine and personalized treatment. Their AI-powered analytics platform analyzes patient genomic and clinical data to identify biomarkers, stratify patient populations, and recommend targeted therapies, improving treatment outcomes and advancing personalized healthcare strategies.

3. **Accelerated Drug Development and Design:**

   Company/Software: BenevolentAI, Atomwise

   Example: BenevolentAI accelerates drug development and design using AI-driven insights in bioinformatics. Their AI platforms predict novel drug targets, simulate molecular interactions, and optimize drug candidates by analyzing biological data, leading to faster discovery and development of therapeutic agents for various diseases.

4. **Predictive Analytics for Disease Prevention:**

Company/Software: 23andMe, Color Genomics

Example: 23andMe employs AI-driven insights in bioinformatics for predictive analytics in disease prevention. Their AI algorithms analyze genetic predispositions, environmental factors, and lifestyle data to predict disease risks, empowering individuals to adopt preventive measures and enabling early intervention strategies for improved health outcomes.

5. **Bioinformatics Tools and Computational Modeling:**

Company/Software: QIAGEN Bioinformatics, Illumina BaseSpace

Example: QIAGEN Bioinformatics develops bioinformatics tools and computational models with AI-driven insights. Their platforms integrate genomic, transcriptomic, and proteomic data with AI algorithms to perform advanced data analysis, visualize molecular interactions, and model biological processes, facilitating innovative research in genomics and personalized medicine.

6. **Ethical Considerations and Regulatory Compliance:**

Company/Software: Illumina, Thermo Fisher Scientific

Example: Thermo Fisher Scientific addresses ethical considerations and regulatory compliance using AI-driven insights in bioinformatics. Their AI systems ensure secure handling of genomic data, comply with GDPR and HIPAA regulations, and adhere to ethical guidelines for genetic research and clinical applications, safeguarding patient privacy and data integrity.

7. **Empowering Healthcare Innovation and Research:**

Company/Software: PacBio, 10x Genomics

Example: PacBio empowers healthcare innovation and research with AI-driven insights in bioinformatics. Their AI-driven technologies enable high-resolution genomic profiling, single-cell analysis, and spatial transcriptomics,

> providing healthcare providers and researchers with comprehensive insights into disease biology and advancing precision medicine initiatives.

These examples demonstrate how AI-driven insights in bioinformatics are transforming healthcare by enhancing data-driven discoveries, enabling precision medicine and personalized treatment, accelerating drug development, predicting disease risks, advancing bioinformatics tools and computational modeling, addressing ethical considerations and regulatory compliance, and empowering healthcare innovation and research globally.

8. Ethical and Legal Considerations of AI in Healthcare

Artificial Intelligence (AI) is increasingly integrated into healthcare systems, offering transformative benefits in patient care, medical research, and operational efficiency. However, the adoption of AI in healthcare necessitates careful consideration of ethical and legal implications to ensure responsible deployment and safeguard patient welfare.

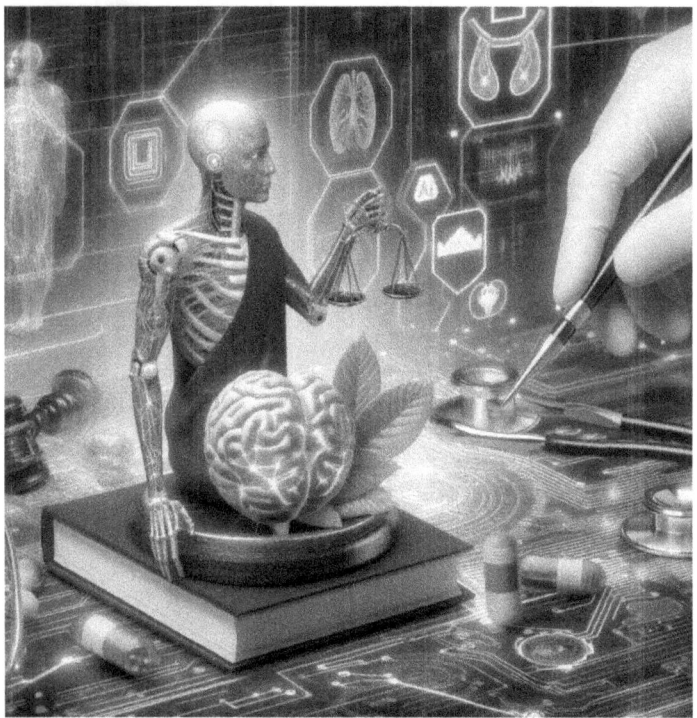

Here's an exploration of key considerations:

1. **Patient Privacy and Data Security:** AI in healthcare relies on vast amounts of sensitive patient data, including medical records, genomic information, and diagnostic images. Ensuring robust data privacy measures and stringent security protocols is essential to protect patient confidentiality and prevent unauthorized access or data breaches. Compliance with regulations such as HIPAA

(Health Insurance Portability and Accountability Act) in the United States and GDPR (General Data Protection Regulation) in Europe is crucial to maintain patient trust and adhere to legal requirements.

2. **Algorithmic Bias and Fairness:** AI algorithms used in healthcare must mitigate biases that could result in unequal treatment or diagnostic inaccuracies across diverse patient populations. Addressing algorithmic bias involves transparent data collection, diverse training datasets, and continuous algorithmic validation to ensure equitable healthcare delivery. Ethical guidelines advocate for fairness, accountability, and transparency (FAT) in AI development and deployment to minimize bias and promote unbiased healthcare outcomes.

3. **Informed Consent and Patient Autonomy:** Implementing AI technologies in clinical settings requires informed consent processes that educate patients about AI's role in treatment, data usage, and potential risks. Respecting patient autonomy involves clear communication of AI's limitations, benefits, and alternatives to enable patients to make informed decisions regarding their healthcare. Upholding ethical standards ensures that patients retain control over their medical information and treatment choices in AI-driven healthcare environments.

4. **Clinical Decision Support and Liability:** AI-enabled clinical decision support systems assist healthcare providers in diagnostic interpretation, treatment planning, and patient management. Clarifying legal responsibilities and liability for AI-driven recommendations or decisions is essential to navigate potential conflicts between AI-generated insights and clinical judgment. Establishing clear guidelines and protocols for integrating AI into medical practice promotes accountability, enhances decision-making processes, and mitigates legal risks associated with AI-driven healthcare interventions.

5. **Professional Standards and Training:** Healthcare professionals utilizing AI technologies require

specialized training to interpret AI-generated insights, maintain clinical competence, and uphold ethical standards in patient care. Integrating AI education into healthcare curricula ensures that clinicians understand AI's capabilities, limitations, and ethical implications. Continuous professional development fosters interdisciplinary collaboration, promotes ethical AI practices, and enhances healthcare professionals' readiness to leverage AI effectively in clinical settings.

6. **Regulatory Compliance and Standards:** Regulatory frameworks govern AI applications in healthcare to ensure patient safety, efficacy, and ethical conduct. Regulatory bodies establish guidelines for AI validation, clinical trials, and market approval to assess AI's reliability, performance, and adherence to healthcare standards. Complying with regulatory requirements fosters trust in AI technologies, facilitates responsible innovation, and safeguards public health in evolving healthcare landscapes.

7. **Public Trust and Stakeholder Engagement:** Building public trust in AI-driven healthcare involves transparent communication, stakeholder engagement, and ethical governance of AI applications. Engaging patients, healthcare providers, policymakers, and industry stakeholders in ethical discussions fosters consensus on AI's role in improving healthcare delivery while addressing societal concerns, ethical dilemmas, and potential risks associated with AI adoption.

In summary, ethical and legal considerations are integral to the responsible adoption of AI in healthcare, ensuring that AI technologies uphold patient rights, promote fairness, and comply with regulatory standards. By prioritizing patient privacy, mitigating algorithmic bias, respecting informed consent, and enhancing professional standards, healthcare organizations can harness AI's transformative potential to advance patient-centered care, enhance clinical outcomes, and uphold ethical principles in AI-driven healthcare innovation.

8.1 Ethical Implications of AI in Medicine

Artificial Intelligence (AI) is revolutionizing the healthcare industry, offering immense potential to improve patient outcomes, streamline operations, and advance medical research.

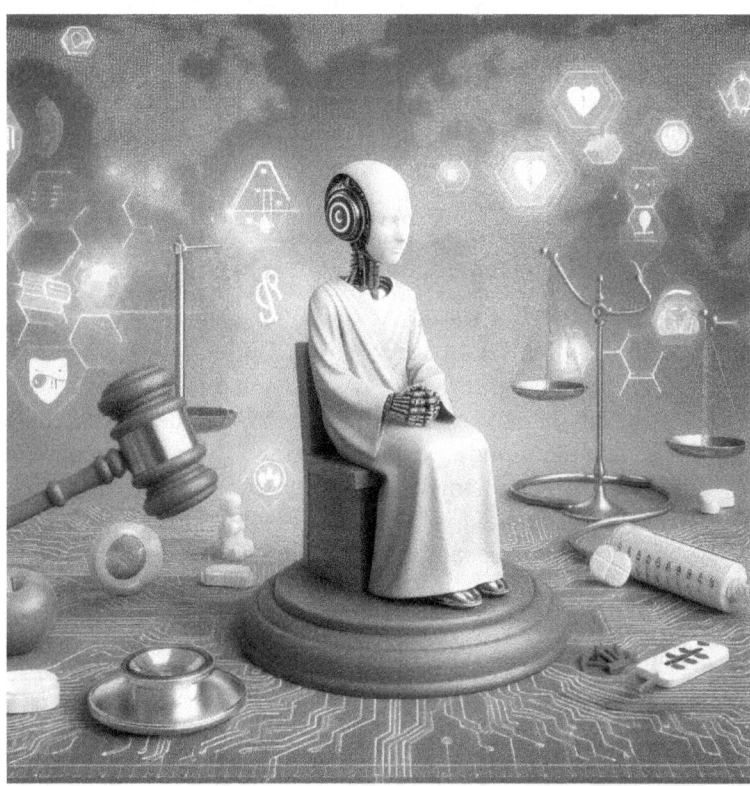

However, the integration of AI in medicine raises significant ethical considerations that must be carefully addressed to ensure responsible and ethical deployment. Here are key ethical implications:

1. **Patient Privacy and Data Security:** AI in medicine relies on extensive patient data, including medical records, genomic information, and diagnostic images. Ensuring robust data privacy measures is crucial to protect patient confidentiality and prevent unauthorized access or breaches. Ethical practices mandate secure data

storage, encryption protocols, and patient consent for data usage to uphold patient privacy rights and maintain trust in AI-driven healthcare systems.

2. **Algorithmic Bias and Fairness:** AI algorithms may inadvertently perpetuate biases based on factors such as race, gender, or socioeconomic status, impacting diagnostic accuracy and treatment recommendations. Ethical AI development requires transparent algorithmic design, diverse training datasets, and rigorous validation to mitigate bias and promote fairness in healthcare delivery. Ethical guidelines advocate for algorithmic accountability and transparency to ensure equitable healthcare outcomes for all patient populations.

3. **Informed Consent and Patient Autonomy:** Implementing AI technologies in clinical practice necessitates informed consent processes that educate patients about AI's role in treatment decisions, data utilization, and potential risks. Respecting patient autonomy involves transparent communication, providing patients with understandable information about AI systems' capabilities and limitations, and obtaining explicit consent for AI-driven interventions. Upholding ethical standards ensures that patients make informed decisions regarding their healthcare, fostering trust and collaboration in AI-enabled medical settings.

4. **Clinical Decision Support and Professional Responsibility:** AI-powered clinical decision support systems assist healthcare providers in diagnosing conditions, interpreting medical imaging, and recommending treatment options. Ethical considerations encompass the professional responsibility of healthcare providers to critically evaluate AI-generated insights, integrate clinical judgment, and prioritize patient well-being. Ethical guidelines emphasize the importance of maintaining human oversight, ensuring that AI complements rather than substitutes medical expertise, and upholding patient-centered care principles in AI-driven clinical practice.

5. **Quality of Care and Accountability:** AI's influence on healthcare quality raises ethical concerns regarding accountability for AI-generated decisions, diagnostic errors, or treatment outcomes. Ethical AI deployment necessitates continuous monitoring, validation, and transparency in AI algorithms' performance to uphold patient safety and mitigate potential harms. Establishing clear guidelines for AI validation, training, and ongoing evaluation promotes accountability, enhances healthcare quality, and safeguards patient interests in AI-integrated healthcare environments.

6. **Healthcare Equity and Access:** AI has the potential to address healthcare disparities by improving diagnostic accuracy, optimizing treatment protocols, and enhancing healthcare delivery efficiency. Ethical considerations emphasize equitable access to AI technologies, ensuring that vulnerable populations benefit from AI-driven healthcare innovations without exacerbating existing disparities. Ethical guidelines advocate for inclusive AI development, promoting healthcare equity, and minimizing barriers to access for underserved communities through responsible AI implementation strategies.

7. **Regulatory Compliance and Ethical Governance:** Regulatory frameworks and ethical guidelines govern AI applications in medicine to ensure patient safety, efficacy, and ethical conduct. Compliance with healthcare regulations, such as FDA (Food and Drug Administration) approvals for AI-based medical devices, and adherence to ethical standards, such as AMA (American Medical Association) guidelines on AI ethics, are essential to navigate legal complexities and ethical challenges in AI-driven healthcare innovation. Ethical governance frameworks promote transparency, accountability, and responsible innovation in AI adoption to uphold patient welfare and public trust.

In summary, addressing ethical implications is paramount to realizing the full potential of AI in medicine while safeguarding patient rights, promoting healthcare equity, and maintaining ethical integrity in AI-driven healthcare ecosystems. By prioritizing patient privacy, mitigating algorithmic bias, respecting informed consent, and fostering professional accountability, healthcare stakeholders can harness AI's transformative capabilities to advance patient-centered care, enhance clinical outcomes, and uphold ethical standards in the evolving landscape of AI in medicine.

8.2 Privacy and Security Concerns

Artificial Intelligence (AI) holds tremendous promise in transforming healthcare by improving diagnostics, enhancing treatment outcomes, and optimizing operational efficiencies. However, the integration of AI in healthcare raises significant privacy and security concerns that must be carefully addressed to safeguard patient data, uphold ethical standards, and maintain trust in AI-driven healthcare systems.

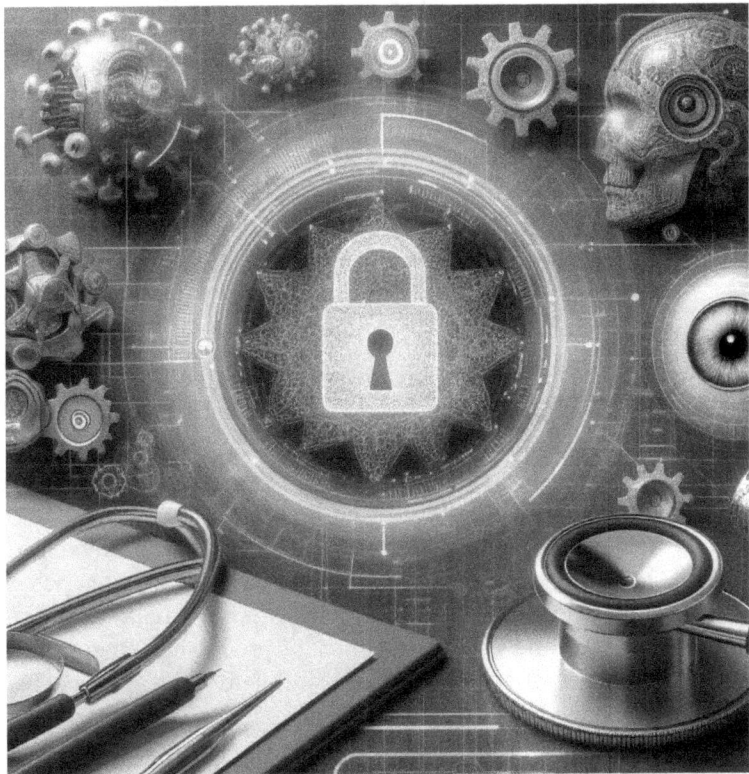

Here are key considerations:

1. **Patient Data Privacy and Confidentiality:** AI in healthcare relies heavily on patient data, including medical records, genomic information, and diagnostic images. Protecting patient privacy is paramount to comply with regulatory requirements (e.g., HIPAA in the

United States) and maintain patient trust. Ethical practices mandate robust data encryption, secure storage solutions, and stringent access controls to prevent unauthorized data breaches or cyberattacks. Implementing anonymization techniques and pseudonymization strategies ensures that patient identities remain protected while leveraging AI for medical insights.

2. **Cybersecurity Risks and Threats:** AI-driven healthcare systems are susceptible to cyber threats, including ransomware attacks, data breaches, and malicious intrusions. Ensuring robust cybersecurity measures involves deploying AI-powered threat detection algorithms to monitor network activities, identify anomalies, and mitigate potential risks proactively. Ethical guidelines advocate for continuous vulnerability assessments, regular security audits, and adherence to cybersecurity best practices to safeguard sensitive patient information and mitigate cybersecurity threats in AI-enabled healthcare environments.

3. **Ethical Use of Patient Data:** Responsible AI deployment requires ethical considerations regarding the collection, storage, and utilization of patient data. Transparency in data practices, including obtaining informed consent from patients for data sharing and AI utilization, is essential to respect patient autonomy and uphold ethical standards. Ethical guidelines promote patient-centric approaches that prioritize data minimization, limit data retention periods, and ensure lawful data processing practices to protect patient rights and mitigate ethical concerns associated with AI-driven healthcare innovations.

4. **Algorithmic Transparency and Accountability:** AI algorithms used in healthcare must exhibit transparency in their decision-making processes to enhance algorithmic accountability and promote trust among healthcare providers and patients. Ethical AI development involves explaining AI-generated insights, disclosing algorithm biases, and providing healthcare professionals with understandable explanations of AI recommendations.

Ensuring algorithmic transparency fosters collaboration between AI systems and healthcare professionals, facilitates informed clinical decision-making, and mitigates concerns regarding the ethical implications of AI in medical practice.

5. **Regulatory Compliance and Legal Frameworks:** Compliance with healthcare regulations (e.g., GDPR in Europe, FDA regulations in the United States) and adherence to ethical guidelines are imperative to navigate legal complexities and ethical challenges in AI integration within healthcare settings. Ethical considerations emphasize adherence to data protection laws, patient rights advocacy, and ethical governance frameworks that prioritize patient welfare, uphold healthcare professionals' ethical responsibilities, and ensure lawful AI deployment practices in healthcare environments.

6. **Trust and Patient-Centered Care:** Building trust in AI-driven healthcare necessitates transparent communication, patient education on AI technologies' roles and limitations, and fostering collaborative partnerships between healthcare providers and patients. Ethical guidelines advocate for promoting patient-centered care principles, respecting patient preferences for AI utilization in medical decision-making, and fostering trustworthiness in AI technologies to enhance patient confidence, satisfaction, and engagement in AI-enabled healthcare services.

7. **Professional Ethics and Responsibility:** Healthcare professionals play a crucial role in maintaining ethical integrity in AI-driven healthcare by upholding professional ethics, adhering to clinical guidelines, and integrating AI technologies responsibly into clinical practice. Ethical considerations encompass healthcare professionals' ethical responsibilities to critically evaluate AI-generated insights, prioritize patient well-being, and advocate for ethical AI use that aligns with patient safety, confidentiality, and privacy requirements.

In summary, addressing privacy and security concerns is essential for the responsible adoption of AI in healthcare, ensuring patient data protection, cybersecurity resilience, ethical AI practices, regulatory compliance, and fostering trust in AI-driven healthcare innovations. By prioritizing patient privacy, enhancing cybersecurity measures, promoting algorithmic transparency, and adhering to ethical guidelines, healthcare stakeholders can harness AI's transformative potential to advance healthcare delivery, improve patient outcomes, and uphold ethical standards in the evolving landscape of AI in healthcare.

8.3 Regulatory and Legal Frameworks for AI in Healthcare

The integration of Artificial Intelligence (AI) in healthcare is poised to revolutionize patient care, clinical decision-making, and operational efficiencies. However, navigating the regulatory and legal landscapes surrounding AI adoption in healthcare is essential to ensure compliance, mitigate risks, and uphold patient safety and ethical standards.

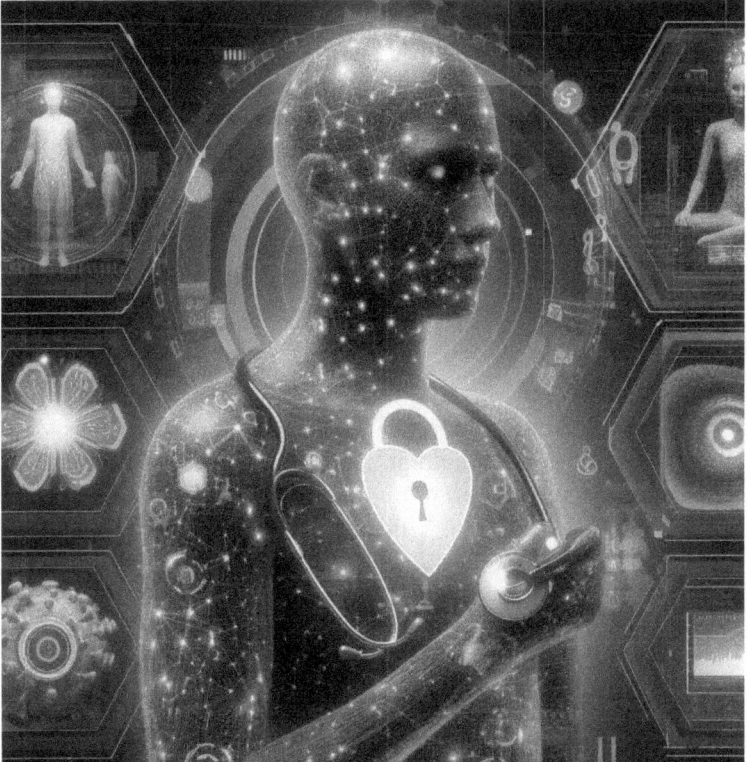

Here are key considerations:

1. **Regulatory Compliance and Governance:** AI technologies used in healthcare must adhere to stringent regulatory standards and governance frameworks to ensure patient safety, data protection, and ethical AI deployment. Regulatory bodies, such as the FDA (Food

and Drug Administration) in the United States and the EMA (European Medicines Agency) in Europe, oversee the approval and regulation of AI-driven medical devices, diagnostics, and treatments. Compliance with regulatory requirements involves rigorous testing, validation of AI algorithms, and adherence to quality assurance protocols to mitigate potential risks associated with AI integration in clinical practice.

2. **Data Privacy and Security:** Protecting patient data privacy and ensuring cybersecurity resilience are paramount in AI-enabled healthcare systems. Compliance with data protection laws (e.g., GDPR in Europe, HIPAA in the United States) mandates secure data storage, encryption techniques, and robust access controls to safeguard sensitive patient information from unauthorized access, data breaches, and cyber threats. Ethical considerations emphasize transparent data practices, patient consent for data utilization, and ethical AI development practices that prioritize patient confidentiality and trust in healthcare AI applications.

3. **Ethical AI Development and Use:** Ethical guidelines govern the development, deployment, and use of AI in healthcare to uphold patient welfare, mitigate biases, and ensure AI algorithms align with clinical best practices and ethical standards. Ethical AI principles advocate for transparency in AI decision-making processes, explainability of AI-generated insights, and accountability in AI-driven clinical decision support systems. Integrating ethical considerations into AI development fosters trust among healthcare providers, patients, and stakeholders, promoting responsible AI use that prioritizes patient safety, autonomy, and equitable healthcare outcomes.

4. **Legal Liability and Responsibility:** Clarifying legal liability and responsibility in AI-driven healthcare environments is crucial to address potential risks, errors, and adverse outcomes associated with AI technologies. Legal frameworks define liability standards for AI

developers, healthcare providers, and stakeholders involved in AI implementation, emphasizing accountability for AI-generated decisions, diagnostic accuracy, and patient outcomes. Establishing clear legal guidelines and liability frameworks mitigates legal risks, enhances patient safety, and ensures equitable access to AI-enabled healthcare services while promoting innovation and technological advancements in medical practice.

5. **Clinical Validation and Evidence-Based Medicine:** Validating AI algorithms through rigorous clinical trials, evidence-based medicine, and real-world data analysis is essential to demonstrate the effectiveness, accuracy, and reliability of AI applications in clinical settings. Regulatory agencies require robust clinical validation studies to assess AI performance, diagnostic accuracy, treatment efficacy, and patient outcomes before widespread adoption in healthcare practice. Ethical considerations promote evidence-based AI deployment that aligns with clinical guidelines, promotes healthcare quality, and enhances patient care delivery while mitigating risks associated with unvalidated AI technologies.

6. **Interoperability and Standards Compliance:** Ensuring interoperability of AI technologies with existing healthcare systems, electronic health records (EHRs), and medical devices requires compliance with interoperability standards, health data exchange protocols, and integration frameworks. Ethical AI integration promotes seamless data interoperability, facilitates information sharing among healthcare providers, and enhances care coordination while respecting patient privacy, data integrity, and regulatory requirements. Standardizing AI interoperability promotes healthcare innovation, optimizes clinical workflows, and supports patient-centered care delivery across healthcare ecosystems.

7. **Continuous Monitoring and Regulatory Updates:** Monitoring AI performance, safety, and regulatory

compliance through post-market surveillance, ongoing monitoring, and regulatory updates is essential to address emerging challenges, technological advancements, and regulatory changes in AI-driven healthcare. Ethical considerations advocate for continuous improvement in AI governance, regulatory oversight, and patient safety initiatives to adapt to evolving healthcare needs, mitigate risks associated with AI technologies, and promote responsible AI innovation in medical practice.

In summary, navigating the regulatory and legal frameworks for AI adoption in healthcare requires compliance with regulatory standards, adherence to data privacy laws, ethical AI development practices, clarity in legal liability, rigorous clinical validation, interoperability standards, and continuous monitoring of AI performance and regulatory updates. By integrating regulatory compliance, ethical principles, and patient-centered care into AI-driven healthcare initiatives, stakeholders can harness AI's transformative potential to improve healthcare delivery, enhance patient outcomes, and promote responsible innovation in the evolving landscape of AI in healthcare.

9. Implementation and Integration of AI in Healthcare Systems

The integration of Artificial Intelligence (AI) in healthcare systems holds significant promise for transforming patient care delivery, clinical outcomes, and operational efficiencies.

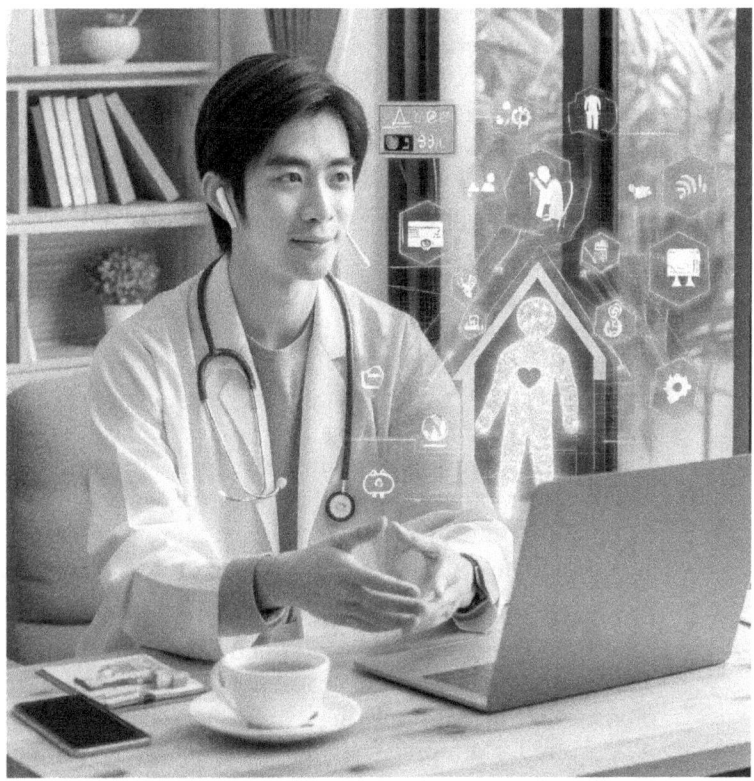

Here are key reasons why the implementation and integration of AI are crucial in healthcare:

1. **Enhanced Clinical Decision-making:** AI empowers healthcare providers to make data-driven clinical decisions by analyzing vast amounts of patient data, including medical records, diagnostic images, and genomic information. AI algorithms can detect patterns, predict disease progression, and recommend personalized treatment plans with higher accuracy than traditional

methods. This capability enhances diagnostic accuracy, supports evidence-based medicine, and improves patient outcomes across diverse medical specialties.

2. **Process Automation and Operational Efficiency:** AI-driven automation streamlines administrative tasks, clinical workflows, and operational processes within healthcare settings. By automating routine tasks such as appointment scheduling, medical transcription, and billing, AI reduces administrative burdens on healthcare professionals, allowing them to focus more on patient care. Improved operational efficiency leads to cost savings, faster patient throughput, and enhanced resource allocation in hospitals, clinics, and healthcare facilities.

3. **Personalized Patient Care and Treatment:** AI enables personalized patient care by analyzing individual health data, genetic information, and lifestyle factors to tailor treatment plans and interventions. Machine learning algorithms can predict patient responses to specific treatments, optimize medication dosages, and identify personalized preventive care strategies. Personalized healthcare improves patient engagement, adherence to treatment regimens, and overall health outcomes by addressing individual patient needs and preferences.

4. **Innovative Medical Research and Development:** AI accelerates medical research and development by analyzing complex biomedical data, identifying disease biomarkers, and discovering novel therapeutic targets. AI-powered platforms facilitate drug discovery, virtual clinical trials, and genomic research, expediting the development of breakthrough treatments and medical innovations. By harnessing AI capabilities, healthcare institutions foster innovation, attract research funding, and contribute to advancements in precision medicine and healthcare delivery.

5. **Predictive Analytics for Public Health:** AI-driven predictive analytics enable proactive public health interventions by forecasting disease outbreaks,

monitoring population health trends, and optimizing resource allocation for healthcare services. AI algorithms analyze epidemiological data, social determinants of health, and environmental factors to identify at-risk populations, prevent disease transmission, and inform public health policies and interventions. Predictive analytics enhance healthcare preparedness, mitigate health disparities, and promote population health management strategies.

6. **Strategic Resource Management and Cost Efficiency:** AI supports strategic resource management in healthcare by optimizing inventory control, predicting patient admission rates, and forecasting healthcare service demands. AI-driven predictive models improve hospital bed management, staff scheduling, and healthcare supply chain logistics, minimizing operational costs and enhancing healthcare service delivery efficiency. Effective resource allocation ensures timely access to care, reduces wait times, and improves healthcare service quality and patient satisfaction.

7. **Ethical and Regulatory Considerations:** Implementing AI in healthcare necessitates adherence to ethical principles, patient privacy regulations (e.g., GDPR, HIPAA), and ethical AI development guidelines. Ethical considerations include transparency in AI decision-making, patient consent for data usage, and mitigating biases in AI algorithms to ensure equitable healthcare delivery. Regulatory compliance ensures patient safety, data security, and legal liability in AI-driven healthcare applications, promoting trust among healthcare providers, patients, and stakeholders.

8. **Collaboration and Interoperability Across Healthcare Ecosystems:** AI integration fosters collaboration among healthcare stakeholders, including hospitals, research institutions, pharmaceutical companies, and technology developers. Interoperable AI systems facilitate seamless data exchange, interoperability standards compliance, and collaborative research initiatives across healthcare

ecosystems. Enhanced collaboration accelerates knowledge sharing, promotes interdisciplinary healthcare approaches, and drives collective efforts toward improving healthcare outcomes and patient care delivery.

In summary, the implementation and integration of AI in healthcare systems are essential to enhance clinical decision-making, automate administrative tasks, personalize patient care, drive medical research innovations, and improve public health outcomes. By embracing AI technologies responsibly, healthcare institutions can optimize operational efficiency, mitigate healthcare challenges, and advance towards a future of precision medicine, equitable healthcare access, and enhanced patient-centered care delivery.

9.1 Strategies for Successful AI Implementation

Successful implementation of Artificial Intelligence (AI) is pivotal for businesses aiming to leverage its transformative potential across various operational domains.

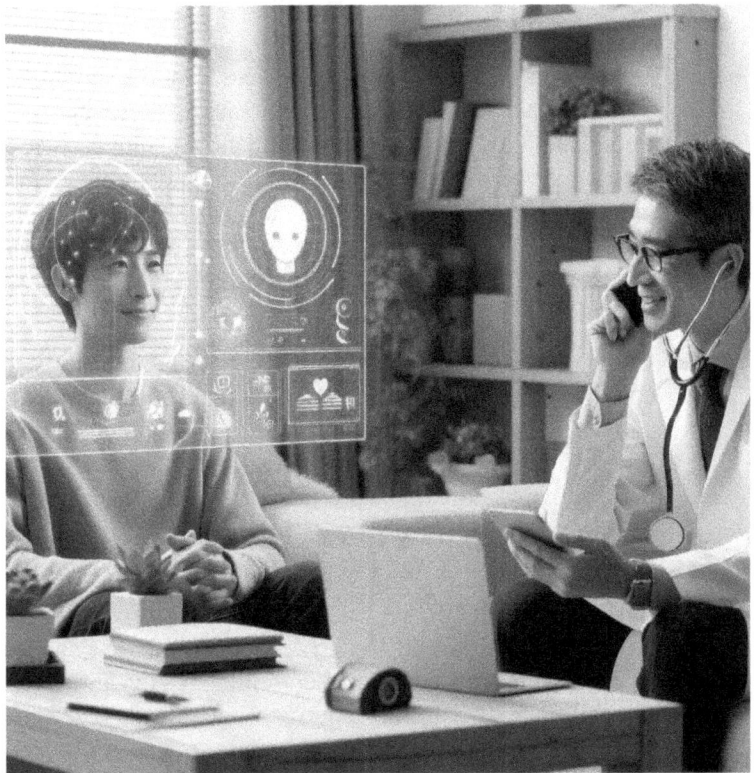

Here are key strategies that organizations should consider to ensure effective AI implementation:

1. **Clear Business Objectives and Alignment:** Define clear and measurable business objectives that AI implementation aims to achieve. Align AI initiatives with overarching business goals such as enhancing customer experience, improving operational efficiency, or driving innovation. Clarity on objectives ensures focused AI deployment and measurable outcomes.

2. **Data Strategy and Preparation:** Develop a robust data strategy that encompasses data collection, quality assessment, integration, and governance. AI relies heavily on data quality and relevance; therefore, organizations should ensure data readiness by cleansing, standardizing, and curating datasets. Establish data pipelines and frameworks to support ongoing data ingestion and preprocessing for AI models.

3. **Investment in Talent and Resources:** Build a skilled AI workforce or collaborate with AI experts to support implementation. Recruit data scientists, AI engineers, and domain specialists capable of developing, deploying, and maintaining AI solutions. Allocate sufficient resources for infrastructure, computing power, and AI tools necessary to support implementation and ongoing operations.

4. **Collaboration and Cross-functional Teams:** Foster collaboration between IT, data science, business units, and stakeholders throughout the AI implementation journey. Form cross-functional teams to ensure diverse perspectives, domain expertise, and alignment with business needs. Encourage open communication, knowledge sharing, and iterative feedback loops to refine AI solutions based on real-world insights.

5. **Proof of Concept and Iterative Development:** Conduct pilot projects or proof-of-concept initiatives to validate AI feasibility and performance in real-world scenarios. Start with small-scale implementations to test AI models, gather feedback, and iterate based on results. Gradually scale successful AI solutions across broader business operations while continuously monitoring performance and optimizing algorithms.

6. **Ethical and Regulatory Compliance:** Prioritize ethical considerations and regulatory compliance when developing and deploying AI solutions. Adhere to data privacy regulations (e.g., GDPR, HIPAA) and ethical guidelines for AI development to protect customer data

and maintain trust. Implement transparent AI practices, mitigate biases, and ensure accountability in AI decision-making processes.

7. **Continuous Monitoring and Evaluation:** Implement robust monitoring mechanisms to assess AI model performance, reliability, and adherence to predefined metrics. Utilize analytics dashboards, AI monitoring tools, and feedback loops to track KPIs, identify issues, and fine-tune algorithms in real time. Regularly evaluate AI impact on business outcomes and adjust strategies as needed to maximize value.

8. **Change Management and Organizational Culture:** Foster a culture of innovation and AI adoption within the organization through change management initiatives. Educate employees about AI benefits, implications, and their roles in supporting AI-driven processes. Encourage adaptability, continuous learning, and experimentation to embrace AI as an enabler of business growth and competitiveness.

9. **Scalability and Future Readiness:** Design AI solutions with scalability and future scalability in mind to accommodate evolving business needs and technological advancements. Plan for integration with existing IT infrastructure, scalability of AI models, and potential expansion into new use cases or markets. Anticipate future AI trends and innovations to maintain competitive advantage and long-term sustainability.

10. **Risk Management and Security Measures:** Implement robust cybersecurity measures and risk management protocols to safeguard AI systems, data assets, and intellectual property. Address potential risks such as data breaches, algorithmic biases, and AI model vulnerabilities through proactive risk assessments, regular audits, and compliance with industry standards.

In conclusion, successful AI implementation requires strategic planning, robust data management, collaboration across teams, ethical considerations, continuous monitoring, and a supportive organizational culture. By following these strategies, businesses can harness AI's transformative potential to drive innovation, enhance decision-making, optimize operations, and maintain competitiveness in the evolving business landscape.

9.2 Integration of AI with Existing Healthcare Systems

The integration of Artificial Intelligence (AI) into existing healthcare systems holds significant promise for enhancing patient care, operational efficiency, and clinical outcomes.

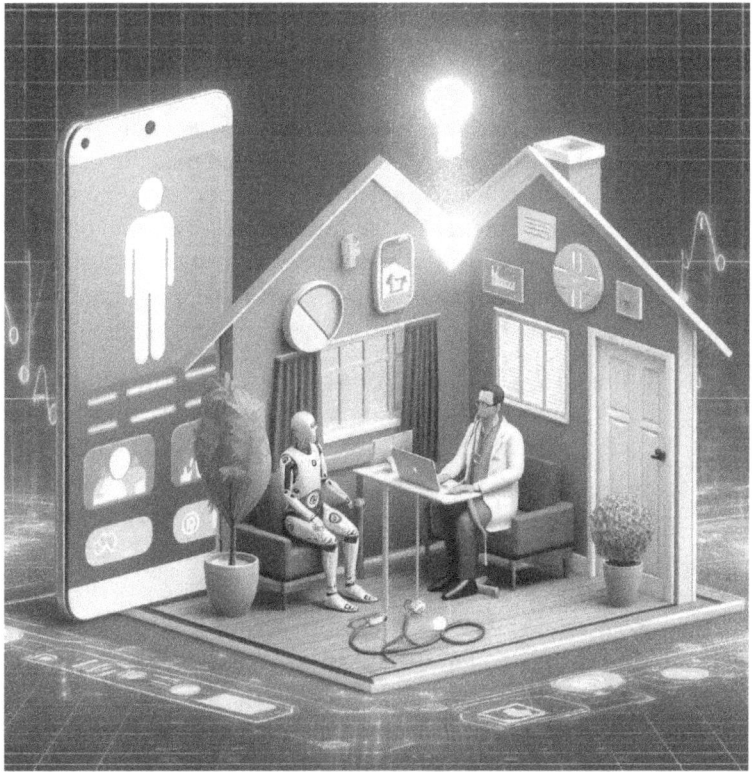

Here are key reasons why integrating AI is crucial for healthcare organizations:

1. **Enhanced Decision-making:** AI enables healthcare providers to make data-driven decisions by analyzing vast amounts of patient data, medical records, and research findings. AI algorithms can uncover patterns, trends, and correlations in data that may not be readily apparent to human clinicians. This capability supports more accurate

diagnostics, personalized treatment plans, and optimized patient outcomes.

2. **Process Automation and Efficiency:** AI-powered automation streamlines administrative tasks, such as scheduling appointments, managing medical records, and processing insurance claims. By automating these routine tasks, healthcare providers can allocate more time to patient care and reduce operational costs associated with administrative overhead.

3. **Improved Patient Experience:** AI technologies like natural language processing (NLP) and machine learning (ML) can enhance patient interactions by providing personalized responses, addressing inquiries, and offering relevant health information. Virtual health assistants powered by AI can offer 24/7 patient support, improving accessibility and responsiveness to patient needs.

4. **Enhanced Clinical Productivity and Innovation:** AI tools augment healthcare professionals' capabilities by performing tasks such as image analysis, pathology screening, and predictive analytics. This allows clinicians to focus on complex cases and innovative research, driving advancements in medical treatments, therapies, and procedural efficiencies.

5. **Predictive Analytics and Insights:** AI enables healthcare organizations to predict patient outcomes, disease progression, and population health trends based on historical data analysis. Predictive analytics support proactive care management, early intervention strategies, and resource allocation optimization, ultimately reducing healthcare costs and improving population health.

6. **Competitive Advantage and Differentiation:** Healthcare organizations leveraging AI gain a competitive edge by offering advanced diagnostics, personalized medicine, and innovative treatment options. By integrating AI-driven solutions, healthcare providers can attract patients seeking cutting-edge care, while

positioning themselves as leaders in medical innovation and quality outcomes.

7. **Scalability and Cost Savings:** AI scalability allows healthcare systems to handle increasing patient volumes, optimize resource utilization, and expand service delivery without compromising quality. AI-driven operational efficiencies, such as reduced diagnostic errors and streamlined workflows, contribute to cost savings and resource allocation optimization.

8. **Risk Mitigation and Regulatory Compliance:** AI enhances healthcare compliance by detecting anomalies, ensuring adherence to medical protocols, and safeguarding patient data privacy. AI systems can monitor for potential risks, cybersecurity threats, and regulatory compliance issues, thereby protecting patient information, organizational reputation, and maintaining trust.

In summary, integrating AI into existing healthcare systems is essential for enhancing clinical decision-making, operational efficiency, patient experience, and innovation in medical care. By leveraging AI technologies responsibly, healthcare organizations can achieve transformative improvements in healthcare delivery, patient outcomes, and overall organizational effectiveness. Embracing AI integration enables healthcare providers to adapt to evolving healthcare demands, drive sustainable growth, and deliver superior care in the modern healthcare landscape.

9.3 AI in Electronic Health Records (EHRs)

The adoption of Artificial Intelligence (AI) in Electronic Health Records (EHRs) has become increasingly important in the healthcare landscape due to its potential to transform patient care, streamline operations, and improve clinical outcomes.

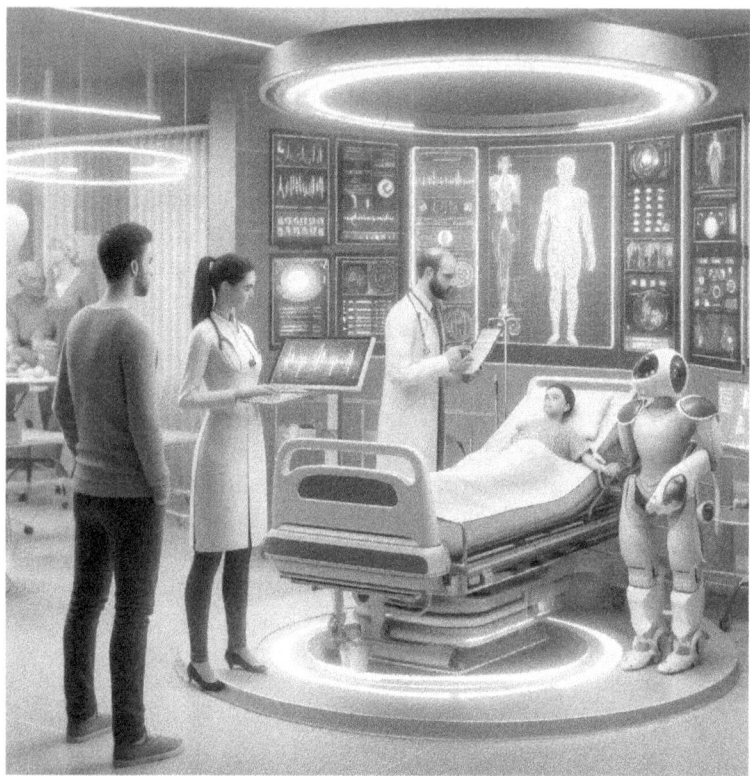

Here are some key reasons why AI adoption in EHRs is crucial:

1. **Enhanced Clinical Decision-making:** AI in EHRs enables healthcare providers to make more informed and timely clinical decisions. By analyzing vast amounts of patient data including medical histories, lab results, imaging reports, and physician notes, AI algorithms can identify patterns, trends, and correlations that may not be readily apparent to healthcare professionals. This

capability enhances diagnostic accuracy, supports treatment planning, and improves patient outcomes.

2. **Automation of Administrative Tasks:** AI-powered automation in EHRs helps streamline administrative workflows and reduce manual tasks. Routine administrative processes such as appointment scheduling, billing, and coding can be automated, allowing healthcare staff to focus more on patient care rather than paperwork. This improves operational efficiency, reduces administrative costs, and enhances overall productivity within healthcare organizations.

3. **Personalized Patient Care:** AI algorithms integrated into EHRs enable personalized medicine by analyzing patient data to tailor treatment plans and interventions. Machine learning models can predict patient risks, recommend personalized therapies, and suggest preventive measures based on individual health profiles and predictive analytics. This personalized approach improves patient engagement, adherence to treatment protocols, and overall patient satisfaction.

4. **Predictive Analytics and Early Intervention:** AI-driven predictive analytics in EHRs help healthcare providers anticipate and mitigate health risks before they escalate. By analyzing historical patient data and monitoring real-time health metrics, AI algorithms can predict potential complications, identify patients at risk of readmission, and recommend proactive interventions. This proactive approach supports preventive care, reduces hospitalizations, and lowers healthcare costs.

5. **Improved Clinical Documentation:** AI technologies enhance the accuracy and efficiency of clinical documentation in EHRs. Natural Language Processing (NLP) algorithms can extract relevant information from unstructured clinical notes, convert speech to text, and suggest standardized documentation templates. This reduces documentation errors, improves data

completeness, and ensures compliance with regulatory requirements.

6. **Research and Population Health Management:** AI in EHRs facilitates population health management and research initiatives by aggregating and analyzing anonymized patient data across large populations. Machine learning algorithms can identify disease trends, conduct epidemiological studies, and evaluate treatment effectiveness on a broader scale. This data-driven approach supports evidence-based medicine, fosters medical research advancements, and informs healthcare policy decisions.

7. **Security and Privacy Enhancements:** AI technologies play a critical role in enhancing the security and privacy of patient data within EHR systems. AI-powered cybersecurity solutions can detect and respond to potential threats, monitor access patterns, and enforce data encryption protocols. By safeguarding sensitive patient information, AI helps healthcare organizations comply with regulatory standards such as HIPAA and GDPR, thereby maintaining patient trust and confidentiality.

8. **Scalability and Integration with Healthcare Systems:** AI-powered EHR systems are scalable and capable of handling large volumes of patient data efficiently. These systems integrate seamlessly with other healthcare IT systems such as telemedicine platforms, diagnostic tools, and wearable devices, ensuring interoperability and continuity of care. This interoperability enhances care coordination, facilitates information exchange among healthcare providers, and supports holistic patient management.

In summary, the adoption of AI in Electronic Health Records (EHRs) is essential for healthcare organizations to enhance clinical decision-making, improve operational efficiency, deliver personalized patient care, and advance medical research. By leveraging AI technologies within EHR systems, healthcare providers can achieve better health outcomes, optimize resource utilization, and meet the evolving demands of modern healthcare delivery.

Examples:

1. **EHR for Enhanced Clinical Decision-making:**

   Company: Google Health

   Example: Google Health's AI-powered EHR system uses natural language processing (NLP) to extract key information from patient records. This data is then analyzed by AI algorithms to provide clinicians with personalized treatment recommendations based on the latest medical research and patient history.

2. **EHR for Automation of Administrative Tasks:**

   Company: Cerner Corporation

   Example: Cerner's AI-powered EHR solutions automate administrative tasks such as appointment scheduling, billing, and coding. Machine learning algorithms streamline workflows by predicting patient scheduling preferences, optimizing resource allocation, and reducing administrative errors.

3. **EHR for Personalized Patient Care:**

   Company: Epic Systems Corporation

   Example: Epic's EHR system incorporates AI to personalize patient care plans based on individual health records and real-time data. Machine learning models analyze patient data to identify personalized treatment options, predict disease progression, and recommend preventive measures tailored to each patient's health profile.

4. **HER for Predictive Analytics and Early Intervention:**

   Company: IBM Watson Health

Example: IBM Watson Health utilizes AI-powered EHR analytics for predictive modeling and early intervention. By analyzing vast amounts of patient data, Watson Health can predict health risks, identify potential complications, and alert healthcare providers to intervene proactively, thereby improving patient outcomes and reducing hospital readmissions.

5. **EHR for Improved Clinical Documentation:**

   Company: Nuance Communications

   Example: Nuance's AI-powered clinical documentation solution for EHRs converts spoken medical dictations into structured patient records using natural language understanding and speech recognition technologies. This improves accuracy, efficiency, and completeness of clinical documentation, enabling clinicians to focus more on patient care.

6. **EHR for Research and Population Health Management:**

   Company: Allscripts Healthcare Solutions

   Example: Allscripts' AI-powered EHR platform supports research initiatives and population health management by aggregating and analyzing anonymized patient data across healthcare systems. Machine learning algorithms identify patterns, trends, and correlations to guide population health strategies, clinical trials, and public health interventions.

7. **EHR for Security and Privacy Enhancements:**

   Company: Microsoft Healthcare

   Example: Microsoft Healthcare integrates AI to enhance security and privacy in EHR systems. AI algorithms monitor access patterns, detect anomalous behavior, and encrypt sensitive patient data to protect against cyber threats and ensure compliance with healthcare regulations like HIPAA.

8. **EHR for Scalability and Integration with Healthcare Systems:**

Company: Siemens Healthineers
Example: Siemens Healthineers' AI-powered EHR solutions are designed for scalability and seamless integration with existing healthcare systems. AI algorithms facilitate interoperability between different healthcare IT platforms, enabling efficient data exchange, collaborative care, and improved operational workflows across healthcare networks.

These examples showcase how leading companies in healthcare and technology are leveraging AI to transform electronic health records management, enhancing clinical decision-making, patient care, administrative efficiency, and overall healthcare outcomes.

9.4 Overcoming Challenges in AI Adoption

The integration of Artificial Intelligence (AI) into healthcare systems presents substantial opportunities for improving patient care, operational efficiency, and medical research. However, several challenges must be addressed to successfully adopt AI in healthcare.

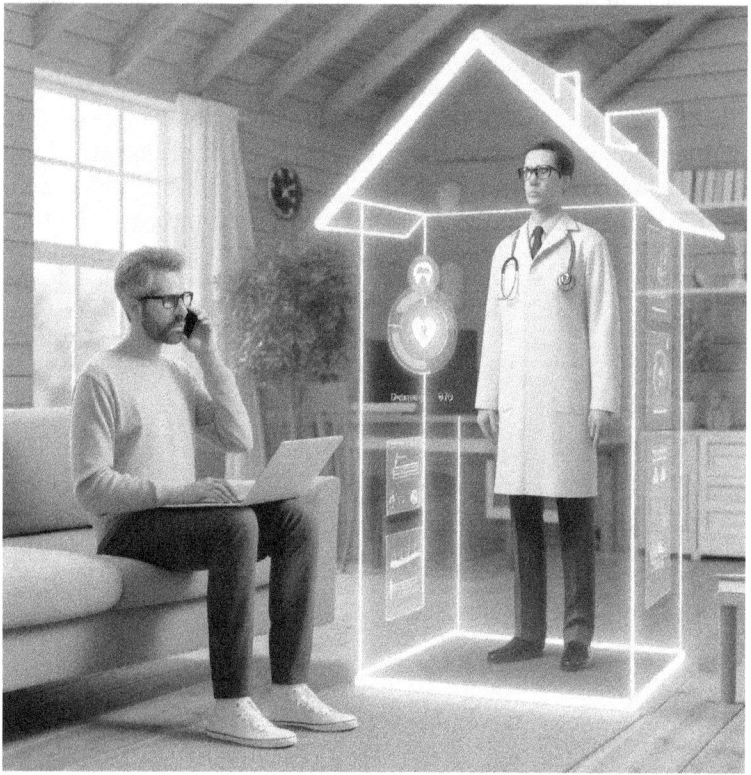

Here are key considerations and strategies to overcome these challenges:

1. **Data Integration and Interoperability:** AI in healthcare relies on access to diverse and comprehensive data sources, including electronic health records (EHRs), medical imaging files, genomic data, and real-time patient monitoring. Challenges often arise due to data silos,

incompatible formats, and varying standards across healthcare systems. Addressing these challenges requires:

- Developing robust data integration frameworks that ensure seamless interoperability across different platforms.
- Implementing standards such as HL7 and FHIR to facilitate data exchange between disparate systems.
- Investing in data cleansing, normalization, and aggregation techniques to ensure data quality and reliability for AI algorithms.

2. **Algorithm Bias and Accuracy:** AI algorithms must be trained on unbiased and representative datasets to avoid perpetuating existing healthcare disparities and inaccuracies. Challenges include:

- Identifying and mitigating biases inherent in training data, particularly related to demographics, socioeconomic factors, and geographic location.
- Implementing algorithm validation and testing protocols to ensure accuracy, reliability, and consistency across diverse patient populations.
- Regularly updating algorithms with new data to enhance performance and adapt to evolving healthcare trends and patient demographics.

3. **Ethical and Regulatory Compliance:** AI adoption in healthcare necessitates adherence to stringent ethical guidelines and regulatory frameworks to safeguard patient privacy, data security, and compliance with healthcare laws such as HIPAA. Challenges include:

- Establishing robust governance structures and ethical guidelines for AI development, deployment, and patient interaction.
- Ensuring transparency in AI decision-making processes and algorithms to foster trust among healthcare providers, patients, and regulatory bodies.

- o Collaborating with regulatory authorities to navigate complex legal landscapes and ensure AI solutions meet compliance standards without compromising innovation.

4. **Integration with Clinical Workflows:** Successful AI adoption requires seamless integration with existing clinical workflows to minimize disruption and enhance efficiency. Challenges include:

- o Customizing AI solutions to align with specific clinical workflows and operational protocols within healthcare settings.
- o Providing user-friendly interfaces and intuitive dashboards that facilitate clinician adoption and acceptance of AI-driven insights.
- o Conducting comprehensive training programs for healthcare professionals to enhance AI literacy and proficiency in utilizing AI tools effectively.

5. **Cost and Resource Allocation:** Implementing AI in healthcare involves significant upfront costs for infrastructure, technology acquisition, and workforce training. Challenges include:

- o Conducting cost-benefit analyses to justify investments in AI technologies based on anticipated improvements in patient outcomes, operational efficiencies, and cost savings.
- o Exploring collaborative funding models, partnerships with technology providers, and government incentives to offset initial investment costs.
- o Optimizing resource allocation to prioritize AI initiatives that deliver maximum value and return on investment (ROI) for healthcare organizations over the long term.

6. **Change Management and Cultural Shift:** Healthcare providers and staff may encounter resistance to change and apprehension about adopting AI technologies due to fear of job displacement or uncertainty about new technological paradigms. Challenges include:

- Implementing robust change management strategies to foster a culture of innovation, continuous learning, and openness to AI-driven transformation.
- Engaging stakeholders through transparent communication, education, and involvement in the AI adoption process to build trust and acceptance.
- Empowering healthcare professionals with the necessary skills and support systems to effectively collaborate with AI technologies and leverage their capabilities to enhance patient care.

7. **Security and Data Privacy Concerns:** AI adoption in healthcare raises concerns about data security, patient confidentiality, and protection against cyber threats. Challenges include:

- Implementing robust cybersecurity measures, encryption protocols, and access controls to safeguard sensitive patient information and AI algorithms.
- Adhering to strict data privacy regulations and industry standards to ensure compliance with healthcare data protection laws (e.g., GDPR, CCPA).
- Enhancing awareness and training among healthcare personnel on cybersecurity best practices and potential risks associated with AI-enabled technologies.

By addressing these challenges proactively and implementing strategic solutions, healthcare organizations can successfully integrate AI into clinical practice, improve patient outcomes, and drive sustainable innovation in healthcare delivery. Embracing AI adoption with a focus on data integrity, ethical considerations, regulatory compliance, and stakeholder engagement will pave the way for transformative advancements in the healthcare industry.

10. Future Trends and Innovations in AI Healthcare

Artificial Intelligence (AI) is poised to revolutionize healthcare by driving transformative advancements in patient care, clinical workflows, and medical research.

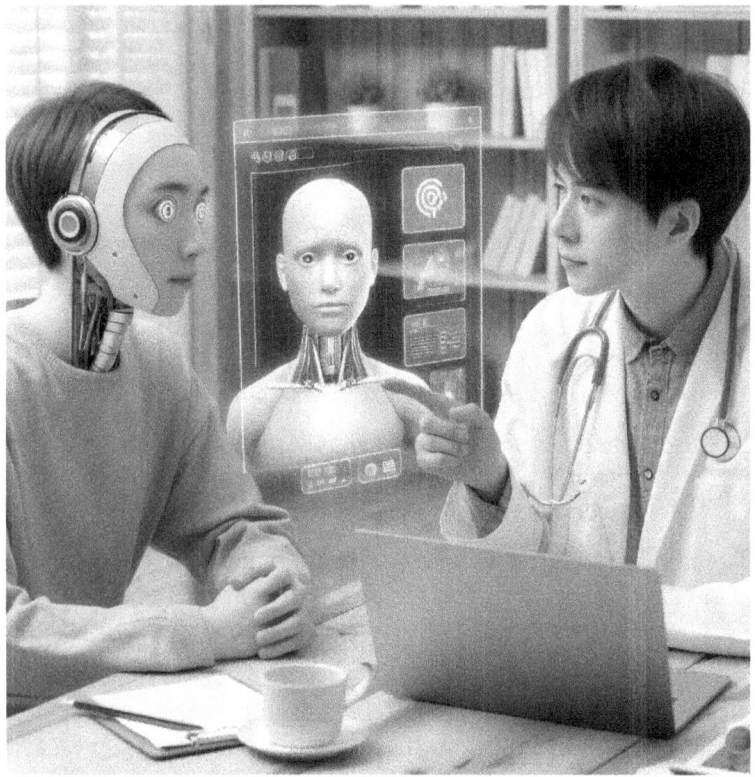

Here are key reasons why AI adoption is crucial in shaping the future of healthcare:

1. Enhanced Diagnostics and Personalized Treatment: AI-powered diagnostic tools are advancing precision medicine by analyzing complex medical data including genetic profiles, imaging scans, and patient records. Machine learning algorithms detect subtle patterns indicative of diseases at early stages, enabling healthcare providers to deliver timely and personalized treatment plans tailored to individual patient needs.

2. Precision Medicine and Personalized Healthcare: AI enables the development of precision medicine by analyzing individual patient data to tailor treatments based on genetic, environmental, and lifestyle factors. This approach enhances treatment efficacy, minimizes side effects, and improves patient outcomes by providing targeted therapies.

3. Telemedicine and Remote Patient Monitoring: AI-powered telemedicine platforms and remote monitoring systems will expand access to healthcare services, especially in underserved areas. AI algorithms can analyze real-time patient data from wearable devices, predict health trends, and alert healthcare providers to intervene early, reducing hospitalizations and improving patient management.

4. Drug Discovery and Development: AI accelerates drug discovery processes by predicting molecular interactions, identifying potential drug candidates, and simulating clinical trials. Machine learning models can analyze vast datasets to uncover new therapeutic targets, streamline clinical trials, and reduce the time and cost involved in bringing new drugs to market.

5. Healthcare Operations Optimization: AI-driven tools optimize hospital and healthcare facility operations by forecasting patient admission rates, allocating resources efficiently, and managing healthcare staff schedules. AI can also improve administrative processes such as billing, coding, and patient record management, enhancing overall operational efficiency.

6. Enhanced Patient Experience and Engagement: AI technologies like natural language processing (NLP) and chatbots improve patient engagement by providing personalized interactions, answering healthcare-related queries, and scheduling appointments. Virtual health assistants powered by AI can offer round-the-clock support, enhancing patient satisfaction and adherence to treatment plans.

7. Predictive Analytics for Disease Prevention: AI algorithms leverage predictive analytics to assess population health trends and individual risk factors. By integrating diverse data sources such as genetic predispositions, lifestyle behaviors, and environmental exposures, predictive models identify high-risk cohorts for chronic diseases, enabling proactive preventive interventions and lifestyle modifications.

8. Ethical Considerations and Regulatory Compliance: As AI becomes more integral to healthcare, addressing ethical concerns such as patient privacy, data security, and algorithm bias becomes crucial. Regulatory frameworks must evolve to ensure AI technologies in healthcare adhere to standards that protect patient rights and maintain trust in healthcare services.

In summary, the future of AI in healthcare promises transformative advancements across diagnosis, treatment, patient care, and operational efficiency. By harnessing AI technologies responsibly, healthcare organizations can improve medical outcomes, enhance patient experiences, and address global health challenges effectively.

Examples:

1. **Enhanced Diagnostics and Personalized Treatment:**

   Company/Software: PathAI, Tempus

   Example: PathAI utilizes AI algorithms to enhance diagnostics and personalize treatment in healthcare. Their AI-powered pathology platform analyzes tissue samples, identifies patterns, and provides pathologists with insights for accurate diagnosis and personalized treatment planning, improving patient outcomes.

2. **Precision Medicine and Personalized Healthcare:**

   Company/Software: Foundation Medicine, SOPHiA Genetics

   Example: Foundation Medicine integrates AI for precision medicine and personalized healthcare. Their AI-driven genomic profiling platforms analyze tumor DNA to identify mutations, predict treatment responses, and match patients with targeted therapies tailored to their genetic profiles, advancing precision oncology and patient care.

3. **Telemedicine and Remote Patient Monitoring:**

Company/Software: American Well (Amwell), BioTelemetry

Example: Amwell leverages AI for telemedicine and remote patient monitoring. Their AI-powered telehealth platform enables virtual consultations, monitors patient vitals remotely, and uses predictive analytics to alert healthcare providers to potential health issues, enhancing access to healthcare services and improving patient outcomes.

4. **Drug Discovery and Development:**

Company/Software: Insilico Medicine, Atomwise

Example: Insilico Medicine applies AI for drug discovery and development. Their AI-driven platforms analyze biological data, simulate molecular interactions, and predict drug efficacy and safety profiles, accelerating the discovery of novel therapeutics for complex diseases and reducing time-to-market for new drugs.

5. **Healthcare Operations Optimization:**

Company/Software: Cerner Corporation, Epic Systems

Example: Cerner uses AI for healthcare operations optimization. Their AI-enabled healthcare management systems analyze patient data, optimize hospital workflows, predict patient admissions, and allocate resources efficiently, enhancing operational efficiency and reducing healthcare costs.

6. **Enhanced Patient Experience and Engagement:**

Company/Software: Conversa Health, Roche Diagnostics

Example: Conversa Health employs AI for enhanced patient experience and engagement. Their AI-driven virtual health assistant platform interacts with patients, provides personalized health education, monitors patient progress, and delivers real-time feedback, empowering patients to manage their health and improving overall engagement.

7. **Predictive Analytics for Disease Prevention:**

> **Company/Software: Ada Health, Google Health**
>
> **Example:** Ada Health utilizes AI for predictive analytics in disease prevention. Their AI-powered symptom checker analyzes patient-reported symptoms, identifies potential health risks, and recommends preventive measures or early intervention strategies, promoting proactive healthcare management and reducing disease burden.

8. **Ethical Considerations and Regulatory Compliance:**

> **Company/Software: IBM Watson Health, Verily Life Sciences**
>
> **Example:** IBM Watson Health addresses ethical considerations and regulatory compliance with AI in healthcare. Their AI systems ensure data privacy, comply with healthcare regulations (such as HIPAA), and adhere to ethical guidelines for AI applications in clinical settings, safeguarding patient confidentiality and maintaining trust in healthcare AI technologies.

These examples illustrate how AI-driven technologies are shaping the future of healthcare by enhancing diagnostics, enabling precision medicine, facilitating telemedicine and remote patient monitoring, accelerating drug discovery, optimizing healthcare operations, improving patient engagement, predicting disease risks, and ensuring ethical compliance in healthcare AI applications.

10.1 Emerging AI Technologies and Innovations

Artificial Intelligence (AI) is revolutionizing the healthcare industry, offering transformative solutions that improve patient care, optimize clinical workflows, and enhance healthcare management.

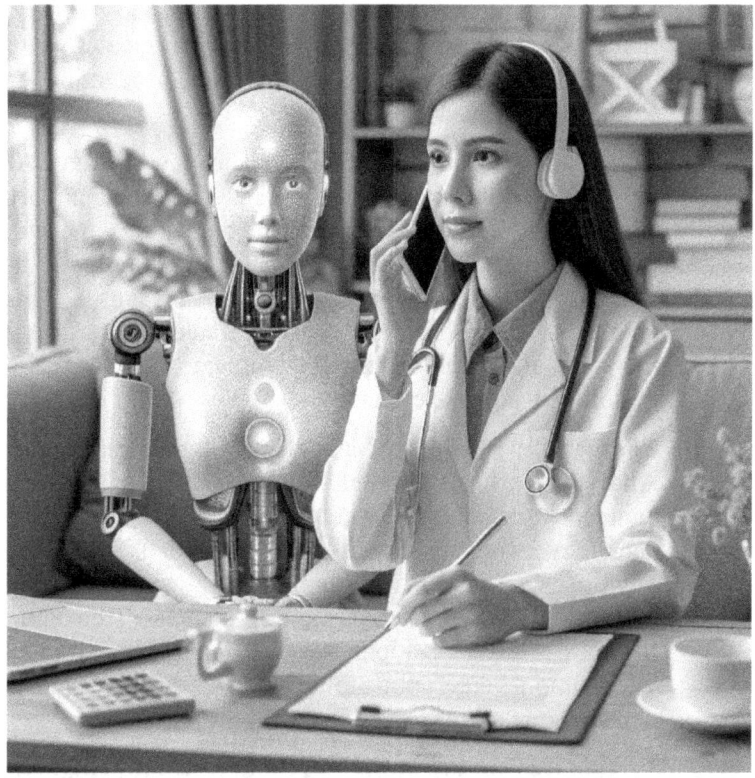

Here are key reasons why the adoption of emerging AI technologies is crucial in shaping the future of healthcare:

1. **Enhanced Diagnosis and Treatment Planning:** AI is revolutionizing healthcare by improving diagnostic accuracy and treatment planning. Machine learning algorithms analyze medical images, genetic data, and patient records to detect patterns and anomalies, enabling earlier and more accurate diagnosis of diseases. AI-driven

decision support systems assist healthcare professionals in selecting optimal treatment plans tailored to individual patient profiles.

2. **Robotics and Surgical Precision:** AI-powered robotics and surgical systems enhance surgical precision, efficiency, and patient safety. Robotics assist surgeons in performing complex procedures with unprecedented accuracy, reducing surgical complications and recovery times. AI algorithms analyze real-time surgical data to optimize procedural outcomes and support continuous learning in surgical practices.

3. **Personalized Medicine and Precision Healthcare:** AI facilitates the advancement of personalized medicine by analyzing vast datasets to identify biomarkers, genetic predispositions, and environmental factors influencing disease susceptibility and treatment response. This approach enables healthcare providers to deliver targeted therapies and interventions, maximizing efficacy while minimizing adverse effects.

4. **Population Health Management and Healthcare Analytics:** AI-driven healthcare analytics platforms aggregate and analyze population health data to improve care delivery and resource allocation. Predictive analytics identify community health needs, monitor disease outbreaks, and forecast healthcare demands, enabling healthcare organizations to implement targeted interventions and optimize healthcare delivery across diverse populations.

5. **Virtual Health Assistants and Remote Monitoring:** AI-driven virtual health assistants and remote monitoring systems enhance patient engagement and care coordination. Natural language processing (NLP) enables virtual assistants to interact with patients, provide real-time health information, schedule appointments, and offer personalized health recommendations, thereby improving patient outcomes and adherence to treatment plans.

6. **Enhanced Patient Engagement and Care Coordination:** AI technologies such as natural language processing (NLP) and virtual health assistants enhance patient engagement by providing personalized health information, facilitating remote consultations, and promoting adherence to treatment plans. AI-driven care coordination platforms improve communication among healthcare teams, ensuring seamless transitions of care and enhancing patient outcomes.

7. **Predictive Analytics for Public Health:** AI enables predictive analytics in public health by analyzing population health data, monitoring disease trends, and predicting healthcare resource demands. AI algorithms detect epidemiological patterns, assess community health risks, and inform public health interventions, contributing to proactive disease prevention and population health management.

8. **Collaborative Research and AI Integration:** AI fosters collaborative research initiatives by facilitating data sharing, interdisciplinary collaborations, and knowledge exchange among healthcare stakeholders. AI integration across healthcare ecosystems promotes innovation, supports evidence-based practices, and drives continuous improvements in clinical care, medical education, and public health initiatives.

In summary, the integration of AI technologies in healthcare promises transformative advancements across diagnosis, treatment, patient care, and operational efficiency. By leveraging AI-driven innovations responsibly, healthcare organizations can enhance clinical outcomes, improve patient experiences, and address global health challenges effectively.

Examples:

1. **Enhanced Diagnosis and Treatment Planning:**

   Company/Software: Aidoc, Zebra Medical Vision

   Example: Aidoc employs AI technologies for enhanced diagnosis and treatment planning in radiology. Their AI-powered platform analyzes medical imaging scans (e.g., CT, MRI) to detect abnormalities, prioritize urgent cases, and assist radiologists in making accurate diagnoses and treatment decisions, improving patient outcomes.

2. **Robotics and Surgical Precision:**

   Company/Software: Intuitive Surgical (da Vinci Surgical System), CMR Surgical (Versius)

   Example: Intuitive Surgical's da Vinci Surgical System integrates AI for robotics and surgical precision. The AI-driven robotic platform enables minimally invasive surgeries, enhances surgical dexterity, and provides real-time feedback to surgeons, improving surgical outcomes and patient recovery times.

3. **Personalized Medicine and Precision Healthcare:**

   Company/Software: Tempus, Deep Genomics

   Example: Tempus applies AI for personalized medicine and precision healthcare. Their AI-driven genomic analysis platform interprets patient data, identifies molecular biomarkers, and recommends targeted therapies tailored to individual genetic profiles, advancing personalized treatment strategies and improving patient responses to treatment.

4. **Population Health Management and Healthcare Analytics:**

   Company/Software: Health Catalyst, Innovaccer

   Example: Health Catalyst utilizes AI for population health management and healthcare analytics. Their AI-powered data analytics platform integrates and analyzes clinical and operational data, identifies at-risk patient populations, predicts health outcomes, and supports proactive interventions to improve population health and reduce healthcare costs.

5. **Virtual Health Assistants and Remote Monitoring:**

> **Company/Software: Babylon Health, Conversa Health**
>
> **Example:** Babylon Health offers AI-driven virtual health assistants and remote monitoring. Their AI-powered chatbot interacts with patients, provides health advice, monitors symptoms remotely, and alerts healthcare providers to potential health issues, enhancing patient engagement and enabling proactive healthcare management.

6. **Enhanced Patient Engagement and Care Coordination:**

> **Company/Software: Lumeon, Vida Health**
>
> **Example:** Lumeon leverages AI for enhanced patient engagement and care coordination. Their AI-driven care pathway management platform automates care coordination tasks, personalizes patient care plans, monitors patient progress, and facilitates communication between healthcare teams and patients, improving care quality and patient satisfaction.

7. **Predictive Analytics for Public Health:**

> **Company/Software: BlueDot, Metabiota**
>
> **Example:** BlueDot uses AI for predictive analytics in public health. Their AI-powered infectious disease surveillance platform analyzes global data (e.g., travel patterns, environmental factors) to predict disease outbreaks, monitor epidemics, and inform public health interventions, enabling early detection and containment of infectious diseases.

8. **Collaborative Research and AI Integration:**

> **Company/Software: NVIDIA Clara, Google DeepMind Health**
>
> **Example**: NVIDIA Clara facilitates collaborative research and AI integration in healthcare. Their AI platform supports medical imaging research, accelerates AI model development, and enables healthcare institutions to

> collaborate on AI-driven innovations in diagnosis, treatment, and patient care, advancing the field of medical AI.

These examples demonstrate how emerging AI technologies are revolutionizing various aspects of healthcare, from diagnosis and treatment planning to surgical robotics, personalized medicine, population health management, virtual health assistants, predictive analytics, patient engagement, and collaborative research, while also addressing ethical considerations and regulatory compliance in healthcare AI applications.

10.2 The Future of AI in Global Health

Artificial Intelligence (AI) is poised to revolutionize global health and healthcare management, offering transformative solutions that enhance patient care, optimize healthcare delivery, and address global health challenges.

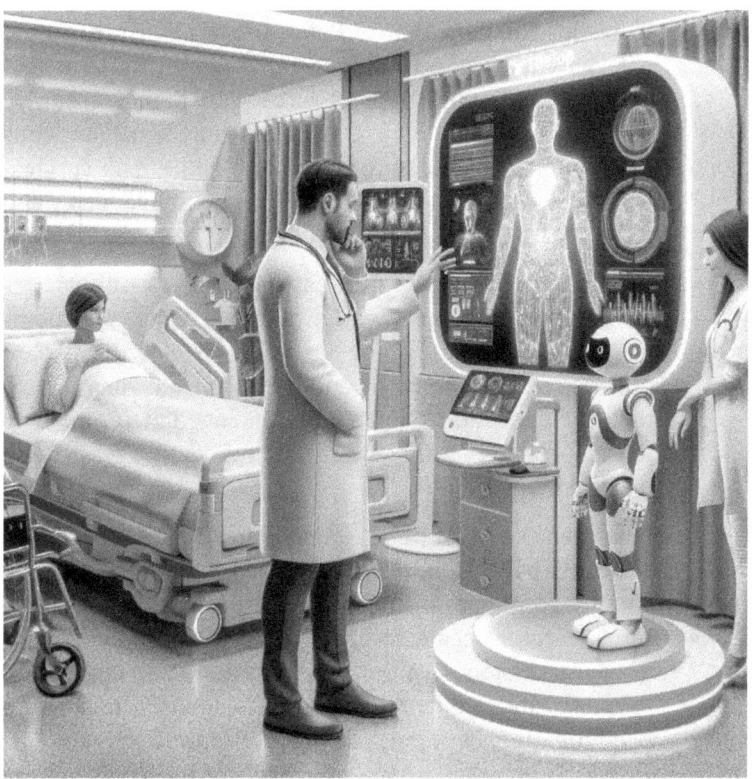

Here are key reasons why the adoption of AI is crucial in shaping the future of global health:

1. **AI-Powered Virtual Assistants and Decision Support Systems**: AI-driven virtual assistants and decision support systems aid healthcare providers in clinical decision-making by analyzing patient data, recommending treatment options, and suggesting personalized care plans based on evidence-based guidelines and patient-specific factors.

2. **Behavioral Analysis and Patient Engagement**: AI tools analyze patient behaviors and preferences to enhance engagement in healthcare management. This includes personalized health coaching, adherence monitoring, and interventions aimed at promoting healthier lifestyles and managing chronic conditions effectively.

3. **Robotic Surgery and Procedural Assistance**: AI enhances surgical precision through robotic systems that can perform complex procedures with higher accuracy and minimal invasiveness. AI algorithms assist surgeons by providing real-time feedback and optimizing surgical workflows, potentially reducing complications and recovery times.

4. **Continuous Medical Education and Training**: AI-powered simulations and virtual reality environments offer immersive training experiences for healthcare professionals. These technologies enable continuous medical education, skill enhancement, and proficiency testing across various specialties and geographic locations.

5. **Healthcare Resource Allocation and Demand Forecasting**: AI algorithms analyze healthcare utilization patterns, demographic trends, and epidemiological data to forecast future healthcare demands. This capability aids policymakers and healthcare administrators in optimizing resource allocation, staffing levels, and infrastructure planning to meet population health needs effectively.

6. **Natural Language Processing (NLP) for Clinical Documentation**: NLP technologies interpret and extract relevant information from clinical notes, electronic health records (EHRs), and medical literature. AI-driven NLP improves the accuracy of medical coding, facilitates information retrieval for research purposes, and enhances interoperability among healthcare systems.

7. **AI in Mental Health Assessment and Therapy**: AI-based tools assist in early detection of mental health disorders through analysis of speech patterns, social

media activity, and other behavioral indicators. Virtual therapists and chatbots provide scalable mental health support, personalized therapy recommendations, and crisis intervention services.

8. **AI Ethics and Bias Mitigation**: As AI applications expand in healthcare, addressing biases in data and algorithms becomes crucial. Ethical guidelines and bias detection tools are essential to ensure fair and equitable AI-driven healthcare outcomes, safeguarding against discrimination and disparities in treatment.

9. **Healthcare Operational Efficiency and Resource Optimization:** AI-driven healthcare management systems streamline administrative tasks, optimize hospital operations, and improve workflow efficiency. Robotic process automation (RPA) reduces administrative burdens, enhances revenue cycle management, and ensures regulatory compliance, enabling healthcare organizations to focus on patient care delivery and quality improvement initiatives.

10. **Clinical Research and Drug Discovery:** AI accelerates drug discovery processes by analyzing vast biomedical datasets, predicting drug interactions, and identifying novel therapeutic targets. Machine learning algorithms expedite preclinical trials, optimize drug formulations, and facilitate drug repurposing strategies, fostering innovation in pharmaceutical research and development.

11. **Collaborative Innovation and Interdisciplinary Research:** AI fosters collaborative research initiatives among healthcare stakeholders, academia, and industry partners. Interdisciplinary collaborations leverage AI technologies to share healthcare insights, validate clinical findings, and translate research discoveries into evidence-based healthcare practices, driving continuous improvements in patient outcomes and healthcare delivery models.

12. **Public Health Management and Disease Surveillance:** AI enhances public health initiatives by predicting disease

outbreaks, monitoring epidemiological trends, and optimizing resource allocation for healthcare interventions. AI-driven predictive analytics enable proactive disease prevention strategies, early detection of health threats, and effective response planning at a global scale.

13. **Operational Efficiency and Healthcare Delivery Optimization:** AI technologies optimize healthcare operations by streamlining administrative tasks, automating routine processes, and improving patient flow management within healthcare facilities. Predictive analytics and AI-driven decision support systems enhance hospital resource utilization, reduce operational costs, and improve overall service delivery efficiency.

14. **Collaboration and Knowledge Sharing:** AI fosters global collaboration among healthcare professionals, researchers, and policymakers by facilitating data sharing, collaborative research efforts, and knowledge exchange across borders. AI-powered platforms support interdisciplinary collaboration, accelerate scientific discoveries, and promote evidence-based healthcare practices worldwide.

In summary, the integration of AI in global health holds transformative potential to enhance diagnostic capabilities, personalize treatment approaches, expand healthcare access, and improve public health outcomes on a global scale. By leveraging AI technologies responsibly, healthcare systems can address global health challenges, improve healthcare delivery efficiency, and advance towards achieving universal health coverage.

Examples:

1. **AI-Powered Virtual Assistants and Decision Support Systems:**

   > **Company/Software: Cerner Corporation, Epic Systems Corporation**
   >
   > **Example**: Cerner's AI-powered virtual assistant, Chatbots, helps healthcare professionals streamline administrative

tasks and provide clinical decision support. It uses natural language processing (NLP) to interpret queries, access patient records, and offer relevant information, enhancing workflow efficiency and patient care quality.

2. **Behavioral Analysis and Patient Engagement:**

Company/Software: Ginger, Woebot Health

Example: Ginger offers AI-driven behavioral analysis and patient engagement tools for mental health. Their platform uses AI to analyze user responses, provide personalized therapy sessions, monitor progress, and engage patients in ongoing mental health support, improving treatment outcomes and patient adherence.

3. **Robotic Surgery and Procedural Assistance:**

Company/Software: Intuitive Surgical (da Vinci Surgical System), CMR Surgical (Versius)

Example: Intuitive Surgical's da Vinci Surgical System integrates AI for robotic surgery and procedural assistance. It enhances surgical precision, minimizes invasiveness, and facilitates complex procedures across various surgical specialties, improving patient safety and recovery outcomes.

4. **Continuous Medical Education and Training:**

Company/Software: HealthStream, SimX

Example: HealthStream utilizes AI for continuous medical education (CME) and training. Their platform delivers personalized learning modules, simulates medical scenarios using AI-powered virtual patients, and provides real-time feedback to healthcare professionals, enhancing clinical skills and knowledge retention.

5. **Healthcare Resource Allocation and Demand Forecasting:**

Company/Software: Qventus, LeanTaaS

Example: Qventus applies AI for healthcare resource allocation and demand forecasting. Their AI-driven platform analyzes real-time data, predicts patient flow, optimizes bed utilization, and suggests staffing adjustments, improving operational efficiency and patient access to care while reducing costs.

6. **Natural Language Processing (NLP) for Clinical Documentation:**

Company/Software: Nuance Communications (Dragon Medical), M*Modal

Example: Nuance Communications' Dragon Medical uses NLP for clinical documentation. It converts spoken words into text, automates medical transcription, and integrates with electronic health records (EHRs), enabling healthcare providers to document patient encounters efficiently and accurately.

7. **AI in Mental Health Assessment and Therapy with AI in Global Healthcare:**

Company/Software: Quartet Health, Mindstrong Health

Example: Quartet Health utilizes AI for mental health assessment and therapy. Their platform combines AI algorithms with clinical expertise to identify mental health conditions early, deliver personalized treatment plans, and monitor patient progress remotely, improving access to mental healthcare and outcomes.

8. **Healthcare Operational Efficiency and Resource Optimization with AI in Global Healthcare:**

Company/Software: SyTrue, Health Catalyst

Example: SyTrue applies AI for healthcare operational efficiency and resource optimization. Their AI platform automates administrative tasks, streamlines revenue cycle management, optimizes supply chain logistics, and improves operational workflows, reducing costs and enhancing healthcare delivery.

9. **Clinical Research and Drug Discovery:**

Company/Software: BenevolentAI, Recursion Pharmaceuticals

Example: BenevolentAI uses AI for clinical research and drug discovery. Their AI-driven drug discovery platform analyzes biomedical data, identifies novel drug targets, predicts drug interactions, and accelerates the development of new therapies for complex diseases, advancing medical research and patient care.

10. **Collaborative Innovation and Interdisciplinary Research with AI in Global Healthcare:**

Company/Initiative: NVIDIA Clara, Google Health

Example: NVIDIA Clara promotes collaborative innovation and interdisciplinary research in healthcare AI. Their AI platform supports medical imaging research, facilitates AI model development, and fosters collaboration among healthcare institutions and researchers to accelerate innovations in diagnosis, treatment, and healthcare delivery.

11. **Public Health Management and Disease Surveillance:**

Company/Software: BlueDot, Metabiota

Example: BlueDot applies AI for public health management and disease surveillance. Their AI-powered platform analyzes global health data, detects disease outbreaks early, models disease spread, and provides actionable insights to public health authorities, enabling proactive response and containment efforts.

12. **Collaboration and Knowledge Sharing:**

Company/Software: UpToDate (Wolters Kluwer), Doximity

> **Example:** UpToDate employs AI for collaboration and knowledge sharing in healthcare. Their AI-powered clinical decision support tool provides evidence-based medical information, fosters collaboration among healthcare professionals, and facilitates knowledge sharing to improve clinical practice and patient care.

These examples illustrate how AI technologies are transforming various aspects of global healthcare, from enhancing patient care and clinical workflows to improving operational efficiency, advancing medical research, and addressing ethical considerations in AI applications.

10.3 Addressing Future Challenges and Opportunities

Artificial Intelligence (AI) is poised to revolutionize healthcare delivery, offering transformative solutions that improve patient outcomes, optimize healthcare operations, and address emerging challenges.

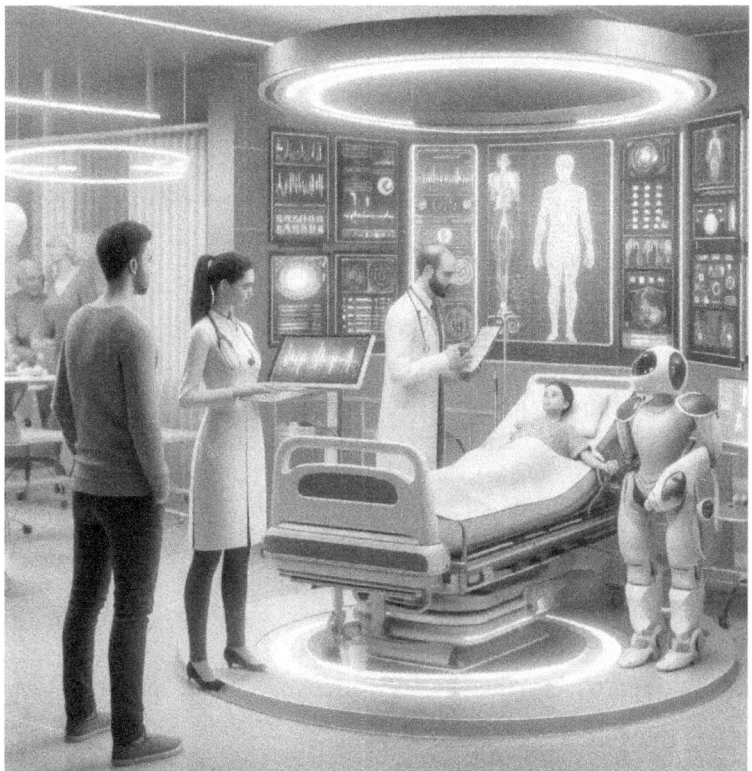

Here are key reasons why addressing future challenges and opportunities in AI-driven healthcare is crucial:
1. **Interoperability and Data Integration**: Ensuring seamless interoperability among healthcare systems and data sources is critical for AI applications. Efforts to standardize data formats, develop robust data sharing protocols, and integrate disparate datasets (such as EHRs,

genomic data, and IoT sensor data) are essential for maximizing the utility of AI in clinical settings.

2. **Cybersecurity and Data Privacy**: Protecting patient data from cyber threats and ensuring privacy is a significant challenge in AI-driven healthcare. Robust cybersecurity measures, encryption protocols, and compliance with data protection regulations (such as GDPR and HIPAA) are necessary to safeguard sensitive health information and maintain patient trust.

3. **Bias Detection and Mitigation**: AI algorithms can inadvertently perpetuate biases present in training data, leading to disparities in healthcare outcomes. Developing methods to detect and mitigate biases in AI models, ensuring fairness and equity in treatment recommendations and diagnostic decisions, is crucial for ethical AI deployment in healthcare.

4. **Patient Empowerment and Informed Consent**: Empowering patients to understand and consent to AI-driven healthcare interventions is essential. Providing clear information about how AI technologies will be used in diagnosis, treatment, and monitoring empowers patients to make informed decisions about their care and enhances trust in healthcare providers.

5. **Regulatory Adaptation and Agile Governance**: Regulatory frameworks must adapt swiftly to the rapid pace of AI innovation in healthcare. Agile governance approaches that balance innovation with patient safety and ethical considerations are needed to facilitate the responsible adoption of AI technologies and ensure compliance with evolving regulatory standards.

6. **Skill Development and Training for Healthcare Professionals**: Integrating AI into clinical practice requires healthcare professionals to acquire new skills in data interpretation, algorithmic understanding, and ethical AI implementation. Continuous education and training programs that equip healthcare providers with AI literacy are essential for maximizing the benefits of AI while minimizing potential risks.

7. **Long-term Impact Assessment and Outcome Measurement**: Evaluating the long-term impact of AI on healthcare outcomes, patient satisfaction, and healthcare costs is critical. Implementing robust metrics and methodologies for outcome measurement and conducting rigorous assessments of AI interventions are necessary to demonstrate value, inform decision-making, and drive continuous improvement in healthcare delivery.

8. **Global Equity in Access and Adoption**: Ensuring equitable access to AI-driven healthcare innovations across regions and socioeconomic groups is a global imperative. Addressing disparities in access to technology, infrastructure, and expertise, and promoting inclusive AI deployment strategies are essential for reducing healthcare inequalities and advancing global health equity.

9. **Ethical AI Research and Responsible Innovation**: Promoting ethical AI research practices, such as transparent reporting of methods and results, engaging diverse stakeholders in decision-making processes, and prioritizing societal benefits over commercial interests, fosters responsible innovation in healthcare. Ethical frameworks and guidelines that emphasize accountability and patient-centricity guide the responsible development and deployment of AI technologies.

These points highlight the multifaceted challenges and opportunities that lie ahead as AI continues to reshape the landscape of global healthcare, emphasizing the importance of ethical considerations, regulatory preparedness, and equitable access in leveraging AI for improved health outcomes.

In summary, addressing future challenges and opportunities in AI-driven healthcare is pivotal for advancing healthcare delivery, improving patient outcomes, and fostering innovation in global health. By harnessing AI capabilities in personalized medicine, predictive analytics, and telemedicine innovations, stakeholders in healthcare can achieve sustainable healthcare solutions and enhance resilience in responding to global health challenges.

11. Case Studies

11.1 Case Study 1: Historical Evolution and Milestones of AI in Medicine by IBM Watson Health

Company/Organization: IBM Watson Health

Overview: IBM Watson Health has been instrumental in advancing the application of artificial intelligence (AI) in medicine, marking significant milestones in the historical evolution of AI technologies within healthcare.

Implementation of AI: IBM Watson Health has implemented AI-driven initiatives across various domains of healthcare, showcasing the evolution and milestones of AI in medicine:

1. **Watson for Oncology:**
   - Problem: Oncologists face challenges in staying updated with vast amounts of medical literature and personalized treatment options for cancer patients.
   - AI Solution: IBM Watson for Oncology leverages natural language processing (NLP) and machine learning algorithms to analyze vast volumes of medical literature, clinical trials, and patient data. It provides evidence-based treatment recommendations tailored to individual patient profiles. This AI system assists oncologists in making informed decisions about treatment plans by presenting relevant information and options in a comprehensible format.

2. **IBM Watson Imaging Clinical Review (formerly Merge PACS):**
   - Problem: Radiologists and clinicians require efficient tools for image interpretation and diagnosis.
   - AI Solution: IBM Watson Imaging Clinical Review integrates AI-powered image analysis into Picture Archiving and Communication Systems (PACS). It

assists radiologists in detecting anomalies, analyzing images for potential abnormalities, and improving diagnostic accuracy. The system uses deep learning algorithms to learn from annotated images and clinical data, enhancing its performance over time.

3. **Drug Discovery and Development:**

- Problem: Pharmaceutical companies face challenges in identifying potential drug candidates and optimizing drug development processes.

- AI Solution: IBM Watson for Drug Discovery accelerates drug discovery by analyzing vast databases of biomedical literature, patents, and molecular data. AI algorithms identify potential drug targets, predict molecular interactions, and optimize drug candidates for specific diseases. This system helps researchers prioritize leads and streamline the drug discovery pipeline, reducing time and costs associated with bringing new therapies to market.

Benefits:

- Enhanced Clinical Decision-Making: AI-powered systems like Watson for Oncology provide oncologists with timely and evidence-based treatment recommendations, leading to more personalized and effective patient care.

- Improved Diagnostic Accuracy: AI in imaging analysis assists radiologists in detecting subtle abnormalities and improving diagnostic precision, potentially reducing missed diagnoses and enhancing patient outcomes.

- Accelerated Drug Discovery: AI-driven drug discovery platforms enable pharmaceutical companies to identify promising drug candidates more efficiently, potentially speeding up the development of new therapies for various diseases.

Challenges and Ethical Considerations:

- Data Privacy and Security: Ensuring that patient data used by AI systems is securely stored and processed in compliance with healthcare regulations (e.g., GDPR, HIPAA).

- Algorithm Transparency: Maintaining transparency in AI algorithms to enable clinicians to understand how decisions are made and ensuring fairness in treatment recommendations across diverse patient populations.

- Integration into Clinical Workflow: Overcoming challenges in integrating AI systems seamlessly into existing clinical workflows without disrupting care delivery or increasing clinician workload.

Conclusion: IBM Watson Health exemplifies the historical evolution of AI in medicine by pioneering AI applications that enhance clinical decision-making, improve diagnostic accuracy, and accelerate drug discovery. Despite challenges in data privacy, algorithm transparency, and workflow integration, IBM Watson Health continues to drive innovation in AI technologies, shaping the future of healthcare delivery and improving patient outcomes globally.

This case study illustrates how AI has evolved from theoretical concepts to practical applications, revolutionizing various aspects of healthcare and laying the foundation for future advancements in medical AI.

11.2 Case Study 2: AI in Medical Imaging and Diagnostics in Healthcare at San Francisco (UCSF) Medical Center, USA

Company/Organization: University of California, San Francisco (UCSF) Medical Center, USA

Overview: UCSF Medical Center has embraced AI technologies to revolutionize medical imaging and diagnostics, aiming to improve accuracy, efficiency, and patient outcomes.

Implementation of AI: UCSF Medical Center has implemented several AI-driven initiatives in medical imaging and diagnostics:

1. **AI-Powered Image Analysis for Radiology:**

   o Problem: Radiologists face challenges in analyzing complex medical images and detecting subtle abnormalities efficiently.

   o AI Solution: UCSF implemented AI algorithms that utilize deep learning and computer vision techniques to analyze medical images such as X-rays, CT scans, and MRIs. These algorithms assist radiologists by automatically highlighting potential areas of concern, quantifying measurements, and providing diagnostic insights. For example, AI can detect early signs of lung cancer on chest X-rays or identify abnormalities in brain MRI scans.

2. **Pathology Image Analysis with AI:**

   o Problem: Pathologists encounter difficulties in processing and interpreting large volumes of tissue samples for cancer diagnosis.

   o AI Solution: UCSF utilizes AI-powered pathology image analysis tools that analyze digital histopathology slides. AI algorithms can detect cancerous cells, grade tumor aggressiveness, and predict patient prognosis based on tissue morphology and biomarker expression patterns. This technology aids pathologists in making accurate diagnoses and treatment recommendations more efficiently.

3. **Integration of AI into Diagnostic Workflows:**

- Problem: Manual review and analysis of medical images are time-consuming and prone to human error.

- AI Solution: UCSF integrates AI into diagnostic workflows to streamline image interpretation and improve diagnostic accuracy. AI algorithms assist radiologists and pathologists by providing quantitative data, comparative analysis with historical cases, and decision support tools that enhance diagnostic confidence and consistency.

Benefits:

- Enhanced Diagnostic Accuracy: AI-driven image analysis improves the detection of abnormalities and early signs of diseases, leading to earlier diagnosis and timely intervention.

- Efficiency Gains: AI automates routine tasks in medical imaging and pathology, allowing healthcare professionals to focus more on complex cases and patient care.

- Improved Patient Outcomes: Early detection and accurate diagnosis facilitated by AI contribute to improved treatment outcomes, reduced morbidity, and enhanced patient satisfaction.

Challenges and Ethical Considerations:

- Data Privacy: Ensuring patient data used for AI analysis is anonymized and securely stored to protect patient confidentiality and comply with privacy regulations (e.g., HIPAA).

- Algorithm Validation: Rigorous validation of AI algorithms to ensure reliability, accuracy, and generalizability across diverse patient populations and imaging modalities.

- Clinical Integration: Effective integration of AI tools into existing clinical workflows without disrupting healthcare operations or adding cognitive burden to healthcare professionals.

Conclusion: UCSF Medical Center's adoption of AI in medical imaging and diagnostics exemplifies the transformative impact of technology on healthcare delivery. By leveraging AI to enhance diagnostic accuracy, streamline workflows, and improve patient outcomes, UCSF demonstrates the potential of AI to revolutionize medical practice. Despite challenges in data privacy, algorithm validation, and workflow integration, ongoing advancements and collaboration with AI developers and healthcare professionals are crucial to maximizing the benefits of AI in medical imaging and diagnostics.

This case study illustrates how AI technologies are reshaping medical imaging and diagnostics, underscoring their potential to advance healthcare delivery and improve patient care outcomes.

11.3 Case Study 3: AI in Predictive Analytics and Disease Prevention at Cleveland Clinic, USA

Company/Organization: Cleveland Clinic, USA

Overview: Cleveland Clinic, renowned for its clinical excellence and innovation in healthcare, has leveraged AI technologies to advance predictive analytics and disease prevention strategies.

Implementation of AI: Cleveland Clinic has implemented several AI-driven initiatives in predictive analytics and disease prevention:

1. **Predictive Analytics for Patient Health Monitoring:**
   - Problem: Healthcare providers need timely insights into patient health trends to intervene early and prevent complications.
   - AI Solution: Cleveland Clinic integrated predictive analytics algorithms into their electronic health records (EHR) system. These algorithms analyze real-time patient data, including vital signs, laboratory results, and medication adherence patterns. AI models predict the likelihood of patients developing specific health conditions such as cardiovascular events, diabetes complications, or sepsis. Healthcare providers receive alerts and risk scores, enabling proactive interventions and personalized preventive care plans.

2. **AI in Population Health Management:**
   - Problem: Public health agencies and healthcare systems require efficient tools for population health management and disease prevention at scale.
   - AI Solution: Cleveland Clinic utilizes AI algorithms to analyze population health data from diverse sources, including EHRs, public health databases, and social determinants of health. AI models identify high-risk populations for diseases such as influenza outbreaks, diabetes epidemics, or community-acquired infections.

Predictive analytics help in allocating resources, implementing targeted interventions, and designing community health programs to mitigate disease risks and improve health outcomes.

3. **Personalized Medicine and Risk Assessment with AI:**
   o Problem: Tailoring treatment plans and preventive strategies to individual patient needs and risk profiles is challenging without comprehensive data analysis.
   o AI Solution: AI algorithms at Cleveland Clinic analyze large datasets of patient demographics, genetic information, lifestyle factors, and medical histories. Machine learning models generate personalized risk assessments for chronic diseases (e.g., cancer, cardiovascular disease) and recommend preventive measures or lifestyle modifications based on individual risk factors. This approach enables proactive management of chronic conditions and reduces the incidence of preventable diseases through personalized interventions.

Benefits:

- **Early Disease Detection:** AI-driven predictive analytics enable early detection of health risks and diseases, facilitating timely interventions and improved patient outcomes.
- **Precision in Preventive Care:** Personalized risk assessments guide targeted preventive strategies, optimizing healthcare resources and reducing healthcare costs.
- **Population Health Management:** AI enhances population health management by identifying at-risk groups and designing proactive interventions to prevent disease outbreaks and improve community health.

Challenges and Ethical Considerations:

- **Data Privacy and Security:** Ensuring the security and confidentiality of patient data used for AI-driven analytics to comply with healthcare regulations (e.g., HIPAA).

- **Algorithm Transparency and Bias:** Addressing biases in AI algorithms to ensure fairness and accuracy in risk assessments and preventive recommendations across diverse patient populations.

- **Integration into Clinical Workflows:** Seamless integration of AI systems into clinical workflows to support healthcare providers in decision-making without disrupting patient care or workflow efficiency.

Conclusion: Cleveland Clinic's adoption of AI in predictive analytics and disease prevention demonstrates the transformative potential of technology in healthcare. By harnessing AI-driven insights for early disease detection, personalized medicine, and population health management, Cleveland Clinic exemplifies how predictive analytics can enhance preventive care strategies, optimize healthcare delivery, and improve overall public health outcomes.

This case study illustrates how AI technologies are applied in predictive analytics and disease prevention, showcasing their role in transforming healthcare by predicting risks, preventing diseases, and improving population health management.

11.4 Case Study 4: Virtual Health Assistants and Chatbots by Babylon Health

Company/Organization: Babylon Health

Overview: Babylon Health is a digital healthcare provider that utilizes AI-driven virtual health assistants and chatbots to enhance patient care accessibility and efficiency.

Implementation of AI: Babylon Health has implemented several AI-driven initiatives through virtual health assistants and chatbots:

1. **AI-Powered Virtual Health Assistant (Babylon Chatbot):**

   o **Problem:** Access to healthcare services can be limited due to geographic barriers, long wait times, and the need for immediate medical advice.

   o **AI Solution:** Babylon Chatbot employs natural language processing (NLP) and machine learning algorithms to interact with patients via chat interfaces. Patients can initiate conversations to receive medical advice, symptom assessment, and guidance on health concerns. The chatbot uses a symptom checker based on medical guidelines and patient input to provide personalized recommendations, such as self-care tips or advice to seek urgent medical attention. This AI-driven solution enhances accessibility to healthcare information 24/7, reducing reliance on traditional in-person or telephone-based consultations.

2. **Telehealth Consultations with AI Integration:**

   o **Problem:** Healthcare providers need efficient tools to conduct remote consultations and follow-ups with patients.

   o **AI Solution:** Babylon Health integrates AI algorithms into telehealth platforms, enabling healthcare professionals to conduct virtual consultations with patients. AI assists in reviewing patient medical records, identifying relevant information, and suggesting treatment options or referrals based on patient history and symptoms discussed during the virtual visit. This approach supports healthcare providers in delivering timely care, managing chronic conditions, and monitoring patient progress remotely.

3. **Health Monitoring and Patient Education:**

- **Problem:** Patients require ongoing monitoring of chronic conditions and access to educational resources for self-management.

- **AI Solution:** Babylon's virtual health assistants support patients with chronic diseases by providing personalized health monitoring reminders, medication adherence alerts, and lifestyle recommendations. AI algorithms analyze patient-reported data and wearable device metrics to track health trends and notify healthcare providers of any significant changes or potential issues. Additionally, the chatbot offers educational content on disease management, healthy living tips, and answers to frequently asked health-related questions, empowering patients to take proactive steps in managing their health.

Benefits:

- **Enhanced Access to Healthcare:** Virtual health assistants provide immediate access to medical advice and information, overcoming barriers of time and distance.

- **Improved Patient Engagement:** AI-driven chatbots engage patients in proactive health monitoring and self-care management, fostering patient empowerment and adherence to treatment plans.

- **Efficiency in Healthcare Delivery:** Telehealth consultations supported by AI streamline the consultation process, optimize healthcare resource utilization, and reduce administrative burdens on healthcare providers.

Challenges and Ethical Considerations:

- **Data Privacy and Security:** Ensuring secure handling of patient data during interactions with AI-driven platforms to maintain patient confidentiality and comply with healthcare regulations.

- **Quality Assurance:** Regular updates and validation of AI algorithms to ensure accuracy, reliability, and alignment with current medical guidelines.

- **Ethical Use of AI:** Mitigating biases in AI algorithms and ensuring transparency in decision-making processes to maintain trust and fairness in patient interactions.

Conclusion: Babylon Health's deployment of AI-powered virtual health assistants and chatbots demonstrates how technology can enhance healthcare delivery by providing accessible, personalized, and efficient patient care solutions. By leveraging AI in telehealth consultations, symptom assessment, and patient education, Babylon Health exemplifies the potential of virtual health assistants to transform healthcare delivery models and improve patient outcomes globally.

This case study highlights how AI-driven virtual health assistants and chatbots are reshaping healthcare delivery, emphasizing accessibility, efficiency, and patient engagement through innovative digital solutions.

11.5 Case Study 5: AI in Drug Discovery and Development at Insilico Medicine

Company/Organization: Insilico Medicine

Overview: Insilico Medicine is a biotechnology company specializing in AI-driven drug discovery and development to accelerate the process of bringing new medicines to market.

Implementation of AI:

1. **AI-Powered Drug Discovery:**

   o Problem: Traditional drug discovery is a lengthy and costly process, often taking years from target identification to clinical trials.

   o AI Solution: Insilico Medicine utilizes deep learning algorithms and generative adversarial networks (GANs) to predict and design novel molecules with desired biological properties. AI analyzes vast databases of chemical compounds, genetic data, and clinical knowledge to identify potential drug candidates. These AI models predict molecular structures that are likely to interact effectively with disease targets, optimizing the selection of lead compounds for further experimental validation. This approach significantly accelerates the early stages of drug discovery, reducing costs and increasing the likelihood of identifying successful drug candidates.

2. **Precision Medicine and Patient Stratification:**

   o Problem: Tailoring treatments to individual patient characteristics and genetic profiles is essential for improving treatment efficacy and reducing adverse effects.

   o AI Solution: Insilico Medicine applies AI algorithms to analyze patient genomic data, biomarkers, and clinical outcomes. Machine learning models identify patient subgroups (stratification) based on genetic variations and disease characteristics to predict responses to specific therapies. This personalized medicine approach helps in selecting patient cohorts for clinical trials, optimizing treatment protocols, and developing targeted therapies that are more effective and safer for individual patients.

3. **Optimization of Clinical Trials:**

- Problem: Conducting efficient clinical trials that yield robust results while minimizing costs and timelines is a challenge in drug development.
- AI Solution: Insilico Medicine integrates AI-driven predictive analytics into clinical trial design and management. AI algorithms analyze historical clinical trial data, patient demographics, and treatment outcomes to optimize trial protocols. This includes predicting patient recruitment rates, identifying potential risks or biases, and optimizing dosing regimens. By leveraging AI insights, the company enhances the efficiency and success rates of clinical trials, accelerating the overall drug development process.

Benefits:

- **Accelerated Drug Discovery:** AI-driven approaches reduce the time and resources required for identifying promising drug candidates, potentially bringing new treatments to patients faster.
- **Precision Medicine:** AI enables personalized treatment strategies based on patient-specific genetic and clinical data, improving treatment outcomes and patient care.
- **Cost Efficiency:** Optimization of drug discovery and clinical trial processes through AI reduces development costs, making innovative treatments more accessible and affordable.

Challenges and Ethical Considerations:

- **Data Privacy:** Ensuring secure handling of patient genomic and health data to protect patient privacy and comply with healthcare regulations.

- **Transparency in AI Algorithms:** Ensuring transparency and reproducibility of AI models used in drug discovery to maintain trust among stakeholders and regulatory bodies.

- **Ethical Use of AI:** Addressing biases in AI algorithms and ensuring equitable access to innovative treatments developed through AI-driven approaches.

Conclusion: Insilico Medicine's application of AI in drug discovery and development exemplifies the transformative impact of technology on advancing healthcare. By harnessing AI for molecular design, precision medicine, and optimizing clinical trials, Insilico Medicine accelerates innovation in pharmaceuticals, paving the way for more effective and personalized therapies that improve patient outcomes globally.

This case study illustrates how AI is revolutionizing drug discovery and development, showcasing its role in accelerating innovation, enhancing precision medicine, and addressing healthcare challenges through advanced technology-driven approaches.

11.6 Case Study 6: AI in Healthcare Operations and Management at Mount Sinai Health System, USA

Company/Organization: Mount Sinai Health System, USA

Overview: Mount Sinai Health System, a prominent healthcare provider in New York City, has implemented AI technologies to optimize operations and management across its network of hospitals and healthcare facilities.

Implementation of AI:

1. **Predictive Analytics for Patient Flow:**

   o Problem: Efficient patient flow management is crucial for reducing wait times, optimizing resource allocation, and enhancing patient satisfaction.

   o AI Solution: Mount Sinai implemented AI-driven predictive analytics models to forecast patient admissions, discharges, and emergency department visits. These models analyze historical data, current patient volumes, and external factors (such as weather and public events) to predict demand patterns. This enables hospital administrators to anticipate surges, adjust staffing levels accordingly, and allocate resources more efficiently. By optimizing patient flow, Mount Sinai improves operational efficiency and enhances the overall patient experience.

2. **AI in Healthcare Supply Chain Management:**

   o Problem: Managing inventory, pharmaceuticals, medical supplies, and equipment across multiple facilities efficiently is challenging without accurate demand forecasting and inventory optimization.

   o AI Solution: Mount Sinai utilizes AI-powered supply chain management systems to streamline inventory management and procurement processes. AI algorithms analyze consumption patterns, expiration dates, and real-time demand data to predict inventory needs accurately.

This ensures that essential supplies are always available without overstocking or shortages, reducing costs and minimizing waste. The system also automates reordering processes, enhancing efficiency and allowing staff to focus on patient care rather than inventory management.

3. **Optimizing Operating Room Scheduling:**
    o Problem: Operating room (OR) scheduling is complex, involving coordination of surgeons, nurses, anesthesiologists, and specialized equipment, while minimizing idle time and maximizing utilization.
    o AI Solution: Mount Sinai implemented AI algorithms to optimize OR scheduling based on historical data, surgical procedure durations, and staff availability. AI analyzes scheduling patterns and patient needs to recommend efficient OR schedules that reduce downtime and enhance utilization rates. By improving OR efficiency, Mount Sinai increases the number of surgeries performed, reduces wait times for procedures, and improves resource utilization across surgical departments.

Benefits:

- **Operational Efficiency:** AI-driven predictive analytics and optimization algorithms improve hospital operations, reducing wait times, optimizing resource allocation, and enhancing overall efficiency.
- **Cost Savings:** Efficient supply chain management through AI reduces inventory costs, minimizes waste, and ensures timely availability of medical supplies and pharmaceuticals.
- **Enhanced Patient Care:** By streamlining operations and improving scheduling, Mount Sinai can increase patient throughput, reduce delays, and provide more timely and effective healthcare services.

Challenges and Ethical Considerations:

- **Data Privacy and Security:** Ensuring that patient data used in AI systems is secure and compliant with healthcare regulations (e.g., HIPAA in the USA).
- **Algorithm Transparency:** Maintaining transparency in AI algorithms to ensure decisions are understandable and accountable to stakeholders.
- **Staff Training and Integration:** Ensuring healthcare staff are trained in AI systems' use and integrating AI tools seamlessly into existing workflows to maximize benefits without disrupting patient care.

Conclusion: Mount Sinai Health System's adoption of AI in healthcare operations and management demonstrates the transformative impact of technology on improving hospital efficiency, patient care quality, and resource utilization. By leveraging AI for predictive analytics, supply chain management, and OR scheduling, Mount Sinai enhances operational performance while optimizing healthcare delivery across its network.

This case study illustrates how AI is pivotal in revolutionizing healthcare operations, driving efficiency, cost-effectiveness, and ultimately improving patient outcomes in large healthcare organizations like Mount Sinai Health System.

11.7 Case Study 7: AI in Genomics and Bioinformatics in Healthcare at Illumina, Inc.

Company/Organization: Illumina, Inc.

Overview: Illumina, Inc. is a global leader in genomics and genetic sequencing technologies, known for its innovative contributions to advancing precision medicine through genomic analysis.

Implementation of AI:

1. **AI-Powered Genomic Data Analysis:**

   o Problem: Analyzing vast amounts of genomic data quickly and accurately is crucial for understanding genetic predispositions, identifying biomarkers, and developing targeted therapies.

   o AI Solution: Illumina has integrated AI algorithms into its genomic data analysis platforms. These algorithms utilize machine learning and deep learning techniques to analyze genomic sequences, identify mutations, detect patterns, and predict potential disease risks. By leveraging AI, Illumina enhances the speed and accuracy of genomic data interpretation, providing clinicians and researchers with actionable insights into patient-specific genetic profiles.

2. **AI in Variant Interpretation:**

   o Problem: Interpreting genetic variants and their clinical significance is complex and time-consuming, requiring specialized knowledge and expertise.

   o AI Solution: Illumina employs AI-driven variant interpretation tools that automate the process of assessing genetic variants. These tools compare genetic data against vast databases of known variants, scientific literature, and clinical guidelines to classify variants based on their potential impact on health. AI algorithms continuously learn from new data, improving accuracy and reliability over time. This accelerates the identification of clinically relevant genetic mutations and supports personalized treatment decisions in clinical settings.

3. **AI-driven Drug Discovery and Development:**
   o Problem: Traditional methods of drug discovery are lengthy and expensive, often resulting in high failure rates.
   o AI Solution: Illumina collaborates with pharmaceutical companies to apply AI in drug discovery processes. AI algorithms analyze genomic data from patients with specific diseases to identify genetic targets and biomarkers associated with drug response. This information enables pharmaceutical researchers to develop targeted therapies tailored to patient genetics, potentially improving treatment efficacy and reducing adverse effects. AI-driven drug discovery accelerates the translation of genomic insights into clinical applications, fostering advancements in precision medicine.

Benefits:

- **Precision Medicine Advancements:** AI enables precise interpretation of genomic data, leading to personalized treatment strategies based on individual genetic profiles.
- **Accelerated Research:** AI-driven insights expedite genetic research and drug discovery, potentially reducing time-to-market for new therapies.
- **Improved Clinical Decision-Making:** Clinicians gain access to timely and accurate genomic information, enhancing diagnostic accuracy and treatment planning.

Challenges and Ethical Considerations:

- **Data Privacy:** Ensuring the security and confidentiality of genomic data used in AI analysis to protect patient privacy.
- **Ethical Use of Genetic Information:** Addressing ethical concerns related to genetic testing, informed consent, and

the implications of genetic insights for individuals and populations.

- **Algorithm Bias:** Mitigating biases in AI algorithms used for genomic analysis to ensure equitable and unbiased healthcare outcomes across diverse populations.

Conclusion: Illumina's integration of AI in genomics and bioinformatics exemplifies the transformative impact of technology on advancing precision medicine. By leveraging AI for genomic data analysis, variant interpretation, and drug discovery, Illumina enhances healthcare delivery, accelerates research innovations, and supports personalized treatment approaches tailored to individual genetic characteristics.

This case study illustrates how AI in genomics and bioinformatics is revolutionizing healthcare by enabling more precise diagnostics, personalized therapies, and innovative approaches to drug development, ultimately improving patient outcomes and advancing the field of precision medicine.

11.8 Case Study 8: Privacy and Security Concerns for AI in Healthcare at Memorial Sloan Kettering Cancer Center, USA

Company/Organization: Memorial Sloan Kettering Cancer Center, USA

Overview: Memorial Sloan Kettering Cancer Center (MSKCC) is a world-renowned cancer treatment and research institution located in New York City. It has implemented AI technologies to enhance cancer diagnosis and treatment processes. However, alongside these advancements, MSKCC faces significant challenges related to privacy and security concerns associated with AI in healthcare.

Implementation of AI:

1. **AI-Powered Imaging Analysis:**
   - Problem: Interpreting complex medical images such as MRI and CT scans requires specialized expertise and can be time-consuming.
   - AI Solution: MSKCC integrated AI algorithms into their imaging systems to assist radiologists in interpreting medical images more accurately and efficiently. These algorithms analyze images to detect subtle patterns and anomalies that may indicate cancerous growth or treatment response. This speeds up diagnosis and enhances treatment planning.
   - Patient Data Protection:
   - Problem: AI systems rely on vast amounts of patient data, including sensitive health information, for training and operation.
   - AI Solution: MSKCC has implemented robust data privacy measures to protect patient information. This includes encryption protocols for data in transit and at rest, stringent access controls, and anonymization

techniques to de-identify patient data used in AI training datasets. Additionally, compliance with HIPAA (Health Insurance Portability and Accountability Act) regulations is strictly followed to ensure patient confidentiality.

2. **Cybersecurity Measures:**

- Problem: AI systems connected to hospital networks are vulnerable to cybersecurity threats such as data breaches and malware attacks.
- AI Solution: MSKCC employs advanced cybersecurity measures to safeguard AI systems and patient data. This includes regular security audits, intrusion detection systems, and staff training on cybersecurity best practices. Additionally, AI systems are designed with built-in security features to detect and mitigate potential threats in real-time.

Benefits:

- **Enhanced Diagnostic Accuracy:** AI-assisted imaging analysis improves the accuracy of cancer detection and treatment planning, leading to better patient outcomes and reduced diagnostic errors.
- **Efficiency Gains:** Faster image analysis allows radiologists to focus more on complex cases and patient care, reducing waiting times and improving overall operational efficiency.
- **Data Security Assurance:** Strict privacy and security measures build patient trust and ensure compliance with regulatory requirements, mitigating the risk of data breaches and protecting patient confidentiality.

Challenges and Ethical Considerations:

- **Patient Consent:** Ensuring informed consent from patients regarding the use of their data in AI systems, especially for research and development purposes.
- **Algorithm Transparency:** Ensuring transparency in how AI algorithms make decisions to maintain

accountability and trust among healthcare providers and patients.

- **Continual Monitoring:** Regular monitoring and updating of AI systems to address evolving cybersecurity threats and ensure data integrity and confidentiality.

Conclusion:

Memorial Sloan Kettering Cancer Center's experience highlights the critical importance of addressing privacy and security concerns in the deployment of AI technologies in healthcare. By implementing robust data protection measures and cybersecurity protocols, MSKCC not only enhances patient care through AI-driven innovations but also upholds patient trust and complies with legal and regulatory requirements. As AI continues to transform healthcare, ongoing vigilance and adaptation of ethical frameworks will be essential to maximize benefits while minimizing risks associated with patient data privacy and security.

11.9 Case Study 9: Overcoming Challenges in AI Adoption in Healthcare at Mount Sinai Health System, USA

Company/Organization: Mount Sinai Health System, USA

Overview: Mount Sinai Health System, a prominent healthcare provider in New York City, has embarked on a journey to integrate AI technologies across its hospitals and clinics. This case study focuses on the challenges faced during the adoption of AI in healthcare and the strategies employed to overcome these hurdles.

Challenges Faced:

1. **Data Integration and Interoperability:**
   - Challenge: Healthcare systems often have disparate data sources and legacy IT systems that hinder seamless integration of AI technologies.
   - Strategy: Mount Sinai Health System invested in developing a robust data infrastructure that could aggregate data from electronic health records (EHR), medical imaging systems, and other sources. They implemented data standardization protocols and employed middleware solutions to ensure interoperability between AI applications and existing healthcare IT systems.

2. **Clinical Acceptance and Workflow Integration:**
   - Challenge: Clinicians may be resistant to adopting AI-driven tools if they perceive them as disrupting established workflows or clinical decision-making processes.
   - Strategy: Mount Sinai engaged healthcare professionals early in the AI implementation process. They conducted extensive training programs and workshops to educate clinicians about the benefits of AI in improving diagnostic accuracy, treatment planning, and patient outcomes. Moreover, they collaborated closely with nurses, physicians, and administrative staff to customize AI

solutions that seamlessly fit into existing workflows without causing disruptions.

3. **Ethical and Regulatory Compliance:**
   o Challenge: Ensuring that AI applications comply with regulatory standards (e.g., HIPAA) and ethical guidelines related to patient privacy and data security.
   o Strategy: Mount Sinai established a dedicated task force comprising legal experts, data privacy officers, and healthcare professionals to oversee AI implementation projects. They conducted thorough risk assessments and privacy impact assessments for each AI application to identify potential ethical concerns and mitigate risks associated with patient data handling. Regular audits and compliance reviews were conducted to ensure adherence to regulatory requirements.

4. **Algorithm Bias and Accuracy:**
   o Challenge: AI algorithms may exhibit biases that could lead to disparities in patient care outcomes, particularly across diverse patient populations.
   o Strategy: Mount Sinai implemented measures to address algorithm bias and improve accuracy in AI predictions. This included diversifying training datasets to better represent the patient demographics served by the healthcare system. They also collaborated with AI developers and researchers to enhance algorithm transparency and accountability, ensuring that clinicians understand the limitations and biases inherent in AI predictions.

Outcome and Benefits:

- **Improved Clinical Decision-Making:** AI integration at Mount Sinai Health System has enhanced the accuracy and speed of clinical decision-making processes. Clinicians can now leverage AI-powered insights to make more informed diagnoses and treatment recommendations.

- **Enhanced Operational Efficiency:** By streamlining data workflows and automating routine tasks, AI has enabled healthcare providers at Mount Sinai to allocate more time and resources to direct patient care, leading to improved patient satisfaction and reduced wait times.

- **Cost Savings:** Through early detection of medical conditions and proactive intervention strategies, Mount Sinai has achieved cost savings by preventing costly complications and hospital readmissions.

Conclusion:

Mount Sinai Health System's experience highlights the importance of addressing challenges systematically to successfully integrate AI into healthcare environments. By focusing on data integration, clinical acceptance, regulatory compliance, and algorithm accuracy, Mount Sinai has overcome initial hurdles and positioned itself at the forefront of AI-driven healthcare innovation. Continuous collaboration with stakeholders and a commitment to ethical AI deployment are essential for realizing the full potential of AI in improving patient outcomes and operational efficiency in healthcare settings.

11.10 Case Study 10: Future Trends and Innovations in AI Healthcare at Cleveland Clinic, USA

Company/Organization: Cleveland Clinic, USA

Overview: Cleveland Clinic, a leading academic medical center, is actively exploring future trends and innovations in AI healthcare to anticipate and address evolving patient care needs.

Focus Area:

Integration of AI in Remote Patient Monitoring

Introduction: Remote patient monitoring (RPM) allows healthcare providers to monitor patients outside of conventional clinical settings, typically at home. AI technologies are increasingly being integrated into RPM systems to enhance monitoring capabilities, improve patient outcomes, and reduce healthcare costs.

Implementation:

1. Enhanced Predictive Analytics for RPM:

- **Challenge:** Traditional RPM systems often rely on basic threshold-based alerts, which may not be sensitive enough to detect subtle changes in patient health status.

- **AI Solution:** Cleveland Clinic has implemented advanced AI algorithms that analyze continuous streams of patient data collected from wearable devices and home monitoring systems. These algorithms detect patterns and trends in vital signs, activity levels, and other health metrics. By leveraging machine learning models, these systems can predict potential health deteriorations or complications before they become clinically apparent. This early warning system enables healthcare providers to intervene promptly, potentially preventing hospitalizations or serious health events.

2. AI-Driven Personalized Medicine:

- **Challenge:** Tailoring treatment plans to individual patient characteristics, including genetic predispositions and lifestyle factors, requires comprehensive data analysis and decision support.
- **AI Solution:** Cleveland Clinic utilizes AI-powered platforms that integrate genomic data, patient histories, and real-time health data to develop personalized treatment plans. Machine learning algorithms analyze vast datasets to identify biomarkers, predict treatment responses, and recommend personalized therapies. This approach not only improves treatment efficacy but also minimizes adverse effects by optimizing drug dosages based on individual patient profiles.

Benefits:

- **Improved Patient Outcomes:** Early detection of health deteriorations through AI-enhanced RPM contributes to proactive healthcare management and better patient outcomes.
- **Enhanced Patient Engagement:** By enabling patients to actively participate in their own care through remote monitoring and personalized medicine, Cleveland Clinic fosters greater patient empowerment and adherence to treatment regimens.
- **Cost Efficiency:** Preventive interventions and personalized treatments resulting from AI-driven RPM systems can lead to reduced healthcare costs by minimizing hospital admissions and emergency room visits.

Challenges and Opportunities:

- **Ethical Considerations:** Ensuring patient consent, data privacy, and confidentiality are maintained throughout RPM and AI-driven healthcare interactions.
- **Regulatory Compliance:** Adhering to regulatory standards such as HIPAA and GDPR in data management and AI application development.

- **Integration with Healthcare Workflow:** Ensuring seamless integration of AI technologies into clinical workflows to minimize disruption and maximize efficiency.

Conclusion:

Cleveland Clinic's initiatives in integrating AI into RPM exemplify the future direction of healthcare, where AI technologies play a pivotal role in transforming patient care through early detection, personalized medicine, and enhanced patient engagement. By addressing challenges and leveraging opportunities in AI healthcare, Cleveland Clinic continues to advance towards delivering more efficient, effective, and patient-centered healthcare solutions. Ongoing research, collaboration with industry partners, and a commitment to ethical AI adoption are essential for realizing the full potential of AI in improving global health outcomes.

12. Popular Software / Systems / Platforms for AI in Healthcare

Following platforms and tools illustrate the diverse applications of AI in healthcare, ranging from clinical decision support and patient monitoring to administrative automation and privacy management.

1. **Cerner HealtheIntent**

   A population health management platform using AI to aggregate and analyze clinical data for insights into patient care pathways and outcomes.

2. **BioMind AI**

   Specializes in AI applications for medical imaging interpretation, aiding in diagnostics and treatment planning through deep learning algorithms.

3. **Olive**

   Description: Provides RPA (Robotic Process Automation) solutions in healthcare, automating administrative tasks like scheduling, billing, and patient record updates.

4. **M*Modal Fluency for Imaging**

   Uses AI-powered speech recognition and natural language processing (NLP) to create structured reports from imaging studies, improving documentation efficiency.

5. **Apervita**

   Offers a secure platform for creating, sharing, and operationalizing AI-driven clinical pathways and protocols within healthcare organizations.

6. **Infermedica**

   Provides AI-driven symptom checker and triage tools for telemedicine platforms, assisting in remote patient assessment and decision-making.

7. **Vocera Engage**

   Integrates AI-enhanced communication tools for healthcare teams, improving collaboration and efficiency in patient care delivery.

8. **Qventus**

   Uses machine learning to predict patient flow bottlenecks and optimize hospital operations, reducing wait times and improving patient outcomes.

9. **Viz.ai**

   AI-powered software for stroke detection and intervention, using deep learning algorithms to analyze CT scans and notify specialists in real-time.

10. **Protenus**

    Utilizes AI for patient data privacy monitoring, detecting and mitigating privacy breaches and unauthorized access in EHR systems.

11. **Watson Health** by IBM

    Comprehensive AI solutions for healthcare analytics, patient insights, and clinical decision support.

12. **DeepMind Health**

    Utilizes AI for patient monitoring, diagnostics, and healthcare management solutions.

13. **Cerner Millennium**

    Includes AI-powered modules for clinical decision support, predictive analytics, and personalized medicine.

14. **Nuance Dragon Medical**

    AI-powered speech recognition software for healthcare documentation and EHR integration.

15. **Zebra Medical Vision**

    AI tools for diagnostic imaging interpretation and early disease detection.

16. **PathAI**

> AI-powered pathology platform for diagnostics and clinical decision support.

17. **Arterys**

> AI-enhanced medical imaging interpretation and analytics platform.

18. **Qventus**

> AI-based software for hospital operations management and patient flow optimization.

19. **Proteus Discover**

> Combines digital medicines and AI to track medication adherence and personalize treatment plans.

20. **Sense.ly**

> Virtual nurse assistant using AI for patient engagement, monitoring, and education.

These platforms and tools illustrate the diverse applications of AI in healthcare, ranging from clinical decision support and patient monitoring to administrative automation and privacy management.